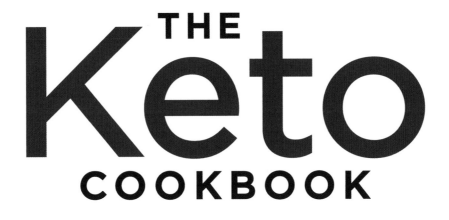

THE Keto COOKBOOK

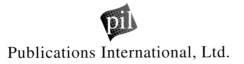

Publications International, Ltd.

Photographs on front cover (bottom) and pages 29, 31, 71 and 149 © copyright Shutterstock.com.

Pictured on the front cover *(top to bottom):* Greek Salad *(page 96)* and Grilled Chicken with Avocado and Spinach *(page 92).*

Pictured on the back cover *(clockwise from top left):* Green Goddess Cobb Salad *(page 94),* Turkey and Veggie Meatballs with Fennel *(page 132)* and Bacon Kale Quiche *(page 22).*

ISBN: 978-1-64558-205-2

Manufactured in China.

8 7 6 5 4 3 2 1

Note: This publication is only intended to provide general information. The information is specifically not intended to be a substitute for medical diagnosis or treatment by your physician or other health care professional. You should always consult your own physician or other health care professionals about any medical questions, diagnosis, or treatment. (Products vary among manufacturers. Please check labels carefully to confirm nutritional values.)

The information obtained by you from this book should not be relied upon for any personal, nutritional, or medical decision. You should consult an appropriate professional for specific advice tailored to your specific situation. PIL makes no representations or warranties, express or implied, with respect to your use of this information.

In no event shall PIL, its affiliates or advertisers be liable for any direct, indirect, punitive, incidental, special, or consequential damages, or any damages whatsoever including, without limitation, damages for personal injury, death, damage to property, or loss of profits, arising out of or in any way connected with the use of any of the above-referenced information or otherwise arising out of the use of this book.

WARNING: Food preparation, baking and cooking involve inherent dangers: misuse of electric products, sharp electric tools, boiling water, hot stoves, allergic reactions, foodborne illnesses and the like, pose numerous potential risks. Publications International, Ltd. (PIL) assumes no responsibility or liability for any damages you may experience as a result of following recipes, instructions, tips or advice in this publication.

While we hope this publication helps you find new ways to eat delicious foods, you may not always achieve the results desired due to variations in ingredients, cooking temperatures, typos, errors, omissions, or individual cooking abilities.

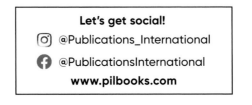

Let's get social!
@Publications_International
@PublicationsInternational
www.pilbooks.com

Contents

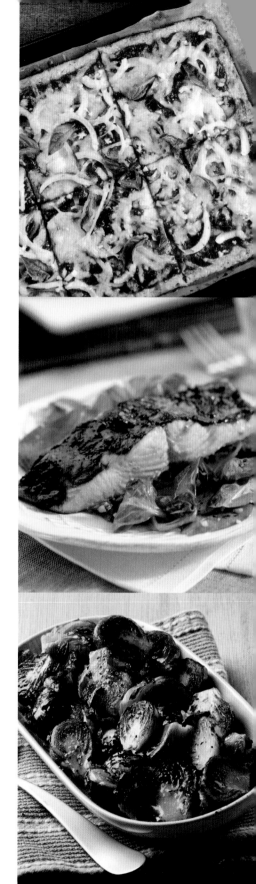

Pictured at right *(top to bottom):* Garlic and Onion Sheet Pan Pizza *(page 78)*, Miso Salmon over Garlicky Spinach *(page 212)* and Brussels Sprouts with Bacon and Butter *(page 214)*.

The Ketogenic Diet and Dieting

The ketogenic diet is hardly new. The idea that fasting could be used as a therapy to treat disease was one that ancient Greek and Indian physicians embraced. "On the Sacred Disease," an early treatise in the Hippocratic Corpus, proposed how dietary modifications could be useful in epileptic management. Hippocrates, a Greek physician called the Father of Modern Medicine, wrote in "Epidemics" how abstinence from food and drink cured epilepsy.

In the 20th century, the first ketogenic diet became popularized in the 1920's and 30's as a regimen for treating epilepsy and an alternative to non-mainstream fasting. It was also promoted as a means of restoring health. In 1921, the ketogenic diet was officially established when an endocrinologist noted that three water-soluble compounds were produced by the liver as a result of following a diet that was rich in fat and low in carbohydrates. The term "water diet" had been used prior to this time to describe a diet that was free of starch and sugar. This is because when carbohydrates are broken down by the body carbon dioxide and water are by-products. When newer, anticonvulsant therapies were established, the ketogenic diet was temporarily abandoned.

In the 1960's the ketogenic diet was revisited when it was noted that more ketones are produced by medium chain triglycerides (MCTs) per unit of energy than by normal dietary fats (mostly long-chain triglycerides) because MCTs are quickly transported to the liver to be metabolized. In research diets where about 60 percent of the calories came from MCT oil, more protein and up to about three times as many carbohydrates could be consumed in comparison to "classic" ketogenic diets. This is why MCT oil is included in some ketogenic diets today.

In the 1950's and 1960's many versions of the ketogenic diet were popularized as high-protein, low-carbohydrate and a quick method of weight loss. Also at this time, the risk factors of excess fat and protein in the diet were criticized for being detrimental to health. Outside of the medical community, the ketogenic diet was not widely recognized for its therapeutic benefits so response to it was sensational in scope.

Then in the 1980's the Glycemic Index (GI) of foods and beverages was revealed that accounted for the differences in the speed of digestion of different types of carbohydrates. This explanation became the springboard for a number of ketogenic diets that were revised from years earlier. By the late 1990's the low-carb craze became one of the most popular types of dieting. Since this time, the original ketogenic diet underwent many refinements and hybrid diets developed.

Variations of the ketogenic diet continued to surface throughout the 20th century since the premise of the ketogenic diet—higher fat and protein and low carbohydrate—was used to treat diabetes and induce weight loss among other applications.

Table 1 summarizes the ketogenic diet basics. Many clinical studies examined their effectiveness and safety and their advantages and drawbacks were identified. These are condensed in **Table 2**.

Table 1

Ketogenic Diet Basics

Generally, the percentages of macronutrients on a ketogenic diet are as follows:

- **Fat** 60 to 75 percent of total daily calories
- **Protein** 15 to 30 percent of total daily calories
- **Carbohydrates** 5 to 10 percent of total daily calories

Both fat and protein have high priority on a ketogenic diet, with non-starchy carbohydrates completing the remaining calories. While calories are not as important on the ketogenic diet as they are for other diets, a closer examination of the contributions of these macronutrients helps to put the amounts into perspective.

If total daily calories were about 2,000, then the percentages of macronutrients on a ketogenic diet would resemble the following amounts:

- **Fat** 60 to 75 percent of total daily calories or about 1,200 to 1,500 calories
- **Protein** 15 to 30 percent of total daily calories or about 300 to 600 calories
- **Carbohydrates** 5 to 10 percent of total daily calories or about 100 to 200 calories

In selecting foods and beverages, think protein and fat first, then non-starchy carbohydrates to complete. Until you truly have a handle on what constitutes low carbohydrates, find a carbohydrate counter to help to keep you in line.

Table 2

Advantages and Drawbacks of Ketogenic Diets

Advantages	Drawbacks
- No calorie counting or focus on portion sizes	- Hard to sustain
- Initial weight loss	- Limited food choices
- After initial transition, hunger subsides	- May lead to taste fatigue
- Improved energy	- Socialization difficult
- Improved blood pressure	- Digestive issues (such as constipation, fatty stool, nausea)
- Improved blood fats: high-density lipoproteins, cholesterol, low-density lipoproteins, triglycerides	- Nutrient deficiencies (such as calcium, vitamins A, C and D, B-vitamins, fiber, magnesium, selenium)
- Reduced blood sugar, C-reactive protein (marker of inflammation), insulin, waist circumference	- Fiber, vitamin and mineral supplements suggested
- Significant short-term weight loss possible	- Increased urination (bladder, kidney contraindications)
	- Diabetes issues
	- Rapid, sizeable short-term weight loss concerning; long-term weight maintenance questionable

Fat In Health and Disease

Fats are essential to the diet and health for many purposes. Fats function as the body's thermostat. The layer of fat just beneath the skin helps to keep the body warm or causes it to perspire to cool the body.

Fat contributes to bile acids, cell membranes and steroid hormones (such as estrogen and testosterone), cushions the body from shock and helps to regulate fluid balance. Too many or too few fats in the diet may influence each of these important body functions.

One of the most important roles of fat in the body is as an energy source, especially when carbohydrates are not available from the diet or are lacking in the body. When people did manual work all day and expended the calories that they consumed, they made good use of carbohydrates and fats in their diet and within their energy stores. Today's laborsaving devices and sedentary lifestyles create less need for excess carbohydrate calories—particularly if they are refined. Even a plant-based diet may be unnecessarily high in refined carbohydrate calories.

Over the years, as humans moved from a plant-based diet toward an animal-based diet, the composition of fatty acids in the American diet switched from monounsaturated and polyunsaturated fats to more saturated fats, which are associated more with cardiovascular disease. A diet that is only filled with saturated fats may not be healthy. Incorporating avocado, fish, nuts, oils and seeds and other foods that contain monounsaturated and polyunsaturated fats into your diet may help to support a healthier proportion of fats in the body for weight maintenance and good health.

Besides cardiovascular disease, excess saturated and trans fats in the human diet are associated with certain cancers, cerebral vascular disease, diabetes, obesity and metabolic syndrome (a collection of conditions that may include abnormal cholesterol or triglyceride levels, excess body fat around the waist, high blood sugar and increased blood pressure that may increase a person's risk of diabetes, heart disease and/or stroke).

The Cholesterol Controversy

Atherosclerosis, or hardening of the arteries, is not a modern disease. Rather, the association between blood cholesterol and cardiovascular disease was recognized as far back as the 1850's.

One hundred years later in the 1950's, cholesterol and saturated fats in the diet were implicated as major risk factors for cardiovascular disease. Then in the 1980's, major US health institutions established that the process of lowering blood cholesterol (specifically LDL-cholesterol) reduces the risk of heart attacks that are caused by coronary heart disease.

Some scientists questioned this conclusion that marked the unofficial start of what's been called the "cholesterol controversy." Studies of cholesterol-lowering drugs known as statins supported the idea that reducing blood cholesterol means less mortality from heart disease. Subsequent statin studies have questioned this association. Other factors aside from dietary cholesterol have since been identified that may lead to elevated blood cholesterol, such as trans fats.

The liver manufactures cholesterol, so reducing cholesterol in the diet should help to reduce blood cholesterol, coronary heart disease and the risk of heart attack. But in some individuals, the liver produces more cholesterol than the body requires and cardiovascular disease may still develop. Accordingly, dietary cholesterol does not necessarily predict cardiovascular disease or a heart attack.

> **WHAT YOU'LL LIKELY END UP WITH IS A SATISFYING EATING PLAN WITH AMPLE PROTEIN, HEALTHY FATS AND MINIMAL CARBOHYDRATES THAT MAY HELP YOU TO FEEL FULL AND LOSE WEIGHT IN THE PROCESS.**

While dietary cholesterol may be a measure for greater cardiovascular risks, cardiovascular disease and heart attacks are also dependent upon such lifestyle and genetic factors as age, diet, exercise, gender, genetics, medication and stress. Reducing hydrogenated fats, saturated fats and trans fats; incorporating mono- and polyunsaturated fats and losing weight to help better manage blood fats are other sensible measures to take.

Longer-term weight management is also a preventative measure in cardiovascular disease. Reducing cholesterol and saturated fat in the diet while integrating foods and beverages with mono- and polyunsaturated fats and oils, dietary fiber, antioxidants and other phytonutrients may lead to a decrease in overall calorie consumption and weight loss and an improvement in overall health.

So What (And How) Should I Eat?

If you want to lose body fat, then the general consensus is that you need to take in fewer calories than you burn for energy. For example, if you're an average woman over 40, decreasing your caloric intake may be a reasonable starting point. If you are of shorter stature and/or very inactive, or you haven't dropped any pounds after a few weeks, you may consider lowering your daily intake of calories by 100-calorie increments until you start seeing weight loss. But don't go much below 1,000 calories without your health care provider's supervision. (And be sure to check with your health care provider before making any major changes to your diet or activity level, especially if you have any serious health problems.)

Another approach to weight loss is the ketogenic diet that does not focus on calories. Instead, the ketogenic diet focuses on the composition of calories from fats, proteins and carbohydrates. Your health care provider may help you determine if this approach to eating and dieting is appropriate for you, so ask your doctor before you begin this or any other diet program.

Table 3

Acceptable Foods, Beverages and Ingredients for Ketogenic Diets

Beverages

- Broth
- Hard liquor
- Nut milks
- Unsweetened coffee, tea
- Water

Eggs

- Egg whites
- Powdered eggs
- Whole eggs

Fats and Oils

- Butter
- Cocoa butter
- Coconut butter, cream and oil
- Ghee
- Lard
- Oils: avocado oil, macadamia nut oil, MCT oil, olive oil and cold-pressed vegetable oils (flax, safflower, soybean)
- Mayonnaise

Fish and Seafood

- Anchovies
- Fish (catfish, cod, flounder, halibut, mackerel, mahi-mahi, salmon, snapper, trout, tuna)
- Shellfish (clams, crab, lobster, mussels, oysters, scallops, squid)

Fruits and Vegetables

- Avocados
- Cruciferous vegetables (broccoli, brussels sprouts, cabbage, cauliflower, kohlrabi)
- Fermented vegetables (kimchi, sauerkraut)
- Leafy greens (bok choy, chard, endive, lettuce, kale, radicchio, spinach, watercress)
- Lemon and lime juice and peel
- Mushrooms
- Non-starchy vegetables (asparagus, bamboo shoots, celery, cucumber)
- Seaweed and kelp
- Squash (spaghetti squash, yellow squash, zucchini)
- Tomatoes (used in moderation in some keto diets)

Dairy Products

- Crème fraîche
- Greek yogurt
- Hard cheese (aged Cheddar, feta, Parmesan, Swiss)
- Whipping cream
- Soft cheese (Brie, blue, Colby, Monterey Jack, mozzarella)
- Sour cream
- Spreadable cheese (cream cheese, cottage cheese and mascarpone)

Meats and Poultry

- Beef (ground beef, roasts, steak, stew meat)
- Goat (leg, loin, rack, saddle, shoulder)
- Lamb (leg, loin, rack, ribs, shank, shoulder)
- Organ meats (heart, kidneys, liver, tongue)
- Poultry with skin (such as chicken, duck, pheasant, quail, turkey)
- Pork (bacon and sausage without fillers, ground pork, ham, pork chops, pork loin, tenderloin)
- Tofu used in moderation in some keto diets)
- Veal (double, flank, leg, rib, shoulder, sirloin)

Non-Dairy Beverages

- Almond milk
- Cashew milk
- Coconut milk
- Soymilk (used in moderation in some keto diets)

Nuts and Seeds

- Nut butters (almond, macadamia)
- Seeds (chia, flax, poppy, sesame, sunflower)
- Whole nuts (almonds, Brazil nuts, macadamia, pecans, hazelnuts, pine nuts, walnuts)

Pantry Items

- Herbs (dried or fresh such as basil, cilantro, oregano, parsley, rosemary and thyme)
- Horseradish
- Hot sauce
- Mustard
- Pepper
- Pesto sauce
- Pickles
- Salad dressings (without sweeteners)
- Salt
- Spices (such as ground red pepper, chili powder, cinnamon and cumin)
- Unsweetened gelatin
- Vinegar
- Whey protein (unsweetened)
- Worcestershire sauce

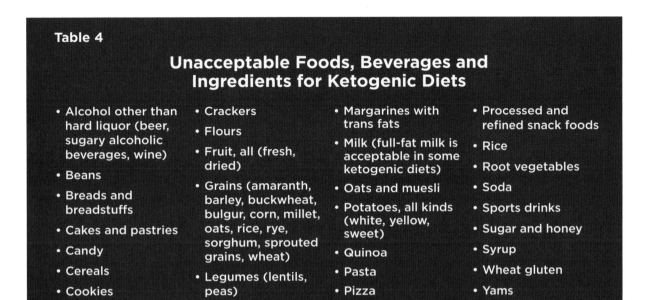

Table 4

Unacceptable Foods, Beverages and Ingredients for Ketogenic Diets

- Alcohol other than hard liquor (beer, sugary alcoholic beverages, wine)
- Beans
- Breads and breadstuffs
- Cakes and pastries
- Candy
- Cereals
- Cookies
- Crackers
- Flours
- Fruit, all (fresh, dried)
- Grains (amaranth, barley, buckwheat, bulgur, corn, millet, oats, rice, rye, sorghum, sprouted grains, wheat)
- Legumes (lentils, peas)
- Margarines with trans fats
- Milk (full-fat milk is acceptable in some ketogenic diets)
- Oats and muesli
- Potatoes, all kinds (white, yellow, sweet)
- Quinoa
- Pasta
- Pizza
- Processed and refined snack foods
- Rice
- Root vegetables
- Soda
- Sports drinks
- Sugar and honey
- Syrup
- Wheat gluten
- Yams

Fats are satisfying because they take longer for the body to digest, and some are converted into ketones for energy. You don't want to skimp on proteins because protein helps maintain and build calorie-burning muscle and also keeps you satiated between meals. Choose protein sources that supply monounsaturated fats and other heart-healthy unsaturated fats; good options include fish, seafood, nuts and seeds. (Fatty fish, such as herring, mackerel, salmon and tuna contain polyunsaturated fats—especially disease-fighting omega-3 fatty acids). You'll need to replace highly processed and refined foods that are full of saturated and trans fats, sugar and refined carbohydrates with minimally processed fiber- and nutrient-rich foods that include non-starchy vegetables.

What you'll likely end up with is a satisfying eating plan with ample protein, healthy fats and minimal carbohydrates that may help you to feel full and lose weight in the process. It's also a plan that may help you to maintain weight loss over time in a modified manner.

If you've ever tried to lose weight before, you know how quickly between-meal hunger may sabotage your best efforts. When your stomach starts rumbling hours before your next meal, it's tempting to grab whatever is available. Often, that "whatever" is some unhealthy packaged snack food or beverage that is loaded with empty calories, sodium, sugars and/or unhealthy fats. Or, if you manage to ignore this hunger, you may become so ravenous at the next meal that you consume far more calories than your body actually needs.

To prevent hunger from spoiling your weight-loss efforts, eat when you are hungry and stop eating when you are full, whether a meal or snack. Try to consume meals and snacks that include a source of hunger-fighting protein and healthy fat, and count your carbs so as not to exceed the daily limit of 20 to 50 grams of non-starchy carbohydrates.

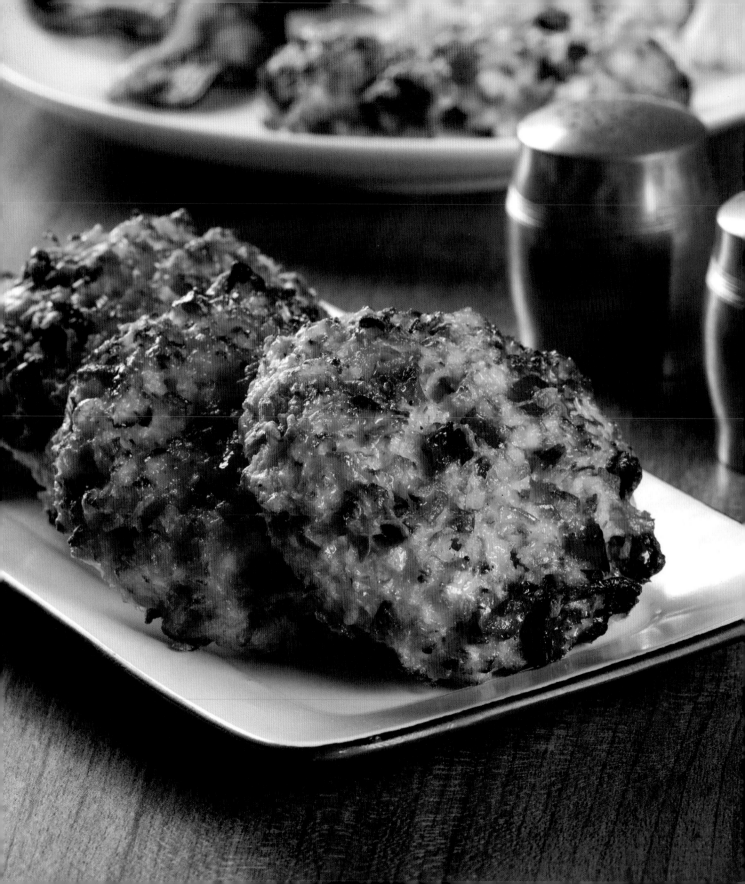

Breakfast

Cauliflower "Hash Brown" Patties
MAKES 8 SERVINGS

1 Place cauliflower in large bowl. Add bacon, onion, bell pepper, egg, almond flour, cheese, chives, salt and black pepper; mix well. Shape mixture into patties; place on baking sheet. Freeze 30 minutes.

2 Preheat oven to 375°F. Bake patties 12 to 15 minutes or until browned.

Nutrients Per Serving (1 patty)
CALORIES 90 **TOTAL FAT** 4g **CARBS** 8g **NET CARBS** 7g
DIETARY FIBER 1g **PROTEIN** 6g

1 package (about 12 ounces) riced cauliflower (fresh or frozen)

4 slices bacon, crisp cooked and crumbled

½ cup finely chopped onion

½ cup finely chopped red and/or green bell pepper

1 egg

⅓ cup almond flour

½ cup (2 ounces) shredded Cheddar cheese

1 tablespoon chopped fresh chives

1 teaspoon salt

½ teaspoon black pepper

6 eggs at room temperature, separated

¼ teaspoon cream of tartar

2 cups almond flour

3½ teaspoons baking powder

½ teaspoon salt

¼ teaspoon garlic powder

6 tablespoons butter, melted and cooled slightly

½ cup finely shredded Asiago cheese

2 tablespoons everything bagel seasoning

Everything Bagels
MAKES 12 BAGELS

1 Preheat oven to 350°F. Spray 12 cavities of doughnut pans with nonstick cooking spray.

2 Place egg whites and cream of tartar in large bowl; attach whisk attachment to stand mixer. Whip egg whites on high speed 2 minutes or until stiff peaks form. Transfer egg whites to medium bowl.

3 Combine almond flour, baking powder, salt and garlic powder in mixer bowl. Add melted butter and egg yolks; mix on medium speed until well blended. Add cheese; mix well.

4 Stir one third of egg whites into almond flour mixture with spatula until well blended (mixture will be very stiff). Gently fold in remaining egg whites until thoroughly blended (mixture may appear mottled). Scoop mixture into large resealable food storage bag; cut off one corner. Pipe about ¼ cup batter into each doughnut cavity. Sprinkle each with ½ teaspoon everything bagel seasoning.

5 Bake about 10 minutes or until bagels are golden brown and set. Cool in pans 2 minutes. Remove to wire rack; serve warm or cool completely.

Everything Bagel Muffins: If you don't have doughnut pans or would prefer to make muffins instead, scoop batter into 12 greased standard muffin pan cups. Sprinkle with bagel seasoning. Bake 15 minutes or until tops are golden brown and toothpick inserted into centers comes out clean.

Nutrients Per Serving (1 bagel)
CALORIES 156   **TOTAL FAT** 13g   **CARBS** 4g   **NET CARBS** 2g
DIETARY FIBER 2g   **PROTEIN** 5g

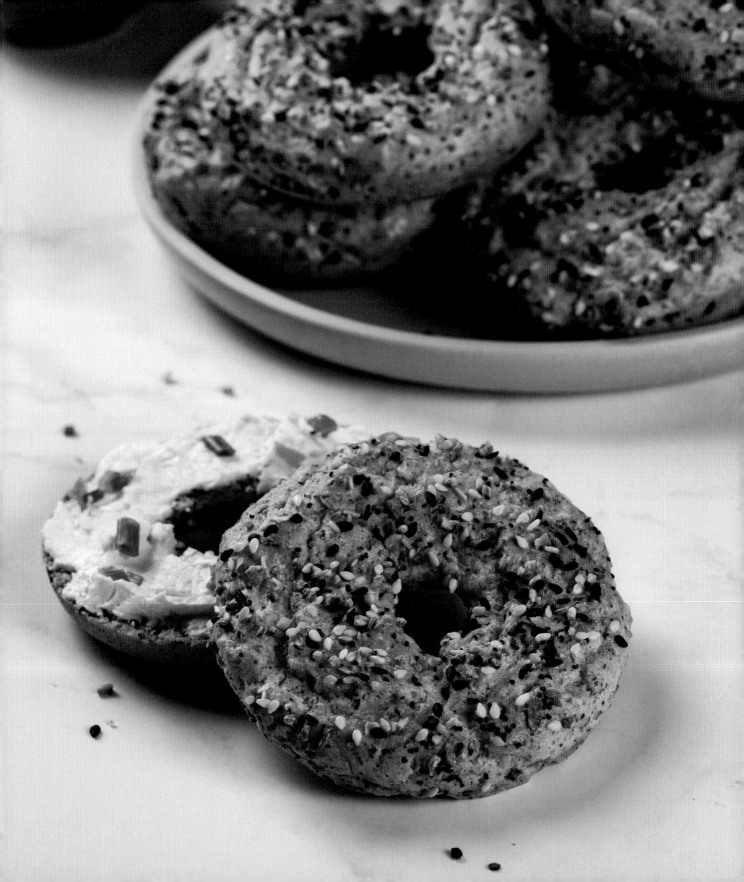

8 eggs
1 cup half-and-half
1 teaspoon Italian seasoning
¾ teaspoon salt
½ teaspoon black pepper
1 package (10 ounces) frozen chopped spinach, thawed and squeezed dry
1¼ cups (5 ounces) shredded Italian cheese blend

Crustless Spinach Quiche
MAKES 6 SERVINGS

1 Preheat oven to 350°F. Spray 8-inch round cake pan with nonstick cooking spray.

2 Whisk eggs, half-and-half, Italian seasoning, salt and pepper in medium bowl until well blended. Stir in spinach and cheese; mix well. Pour into prepared pan.

3 Bake 33 minutes or until toothpick inserted into center comes out clean. Remove to wire rack; cool 10 minutes before serving.

Tip: To remove quiche from pan for serving, run knife around edge of pan to loosen. Invert quiche onto plate; invert again onto second plate. Cut into wedges to serve.

Nutrients Per Serving (1 wedge)

CALORIES 210   **TOTAL FAT** 15g   **CARBS** 6g   **NET CARBS** 5g
DIETARY FIBER 1g   **PROTEIN** 17g

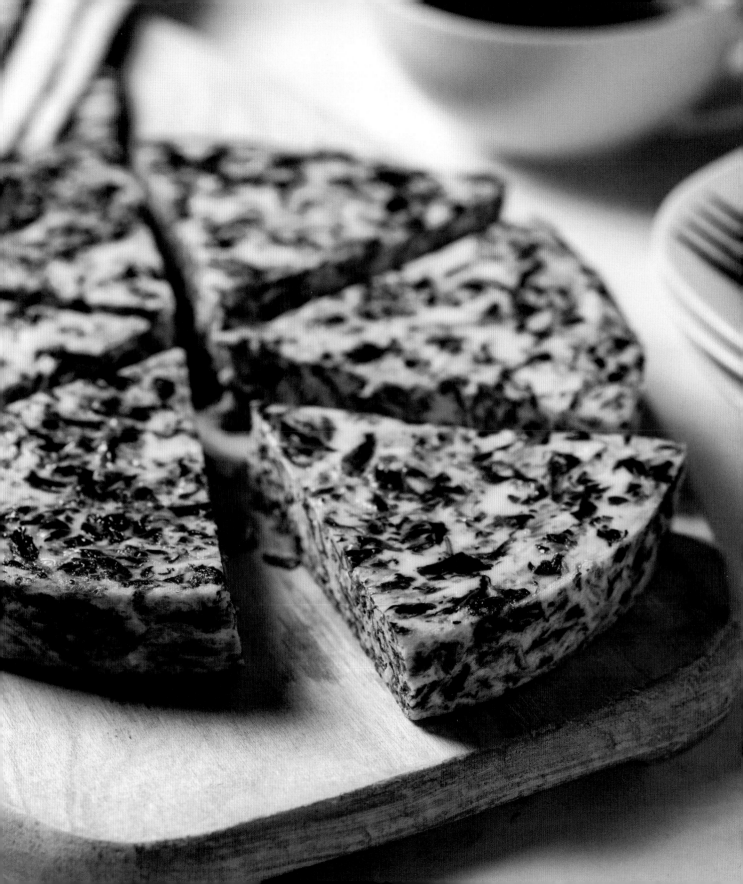

Crust

2 cups riced cauliflower (fresh or frozen)

½ cup shredded Parmesan cheese

1 egg

½ teaspoon salt

⅛ teaspoon ground red pepper (optional)

Filling

1 package (about 12 ounces) bacon, chopped

1 onion, chopped

1 jalapeño pepper, seeded and chopped

2 cloves garlic, minced

1 cup (4 ounces) shredded Cheddar cheese, divided

8 eggs

¾ cup milk

¼ teaspoon salt

Bacon and Egg Breakfast Casserole

MAKES 6 SERVINGS

1 Preheat oven to 400°F. Place cauliflower in medium microwavable bowl; cover with plastic wrap and cut slit to vent. Microwave on HIGH 6 minutes. Remove cover; cool slightly. Press cauliflower with paper towels to remove excess moisture. Add Parmesan cheese, 1 egg, ½ teaspoon salt and red pepper, if desired; mix well. Press onto bottom and up side of 8-inch square baking pan. Bake 15 minutes. Remove from oven. *Reduce oven temperature to 350°F.*

2 Meanwhile, cook bacon in large skillet over medium heat until crisp. Remove with slotted spoon to paper towels to drain. Drain all but 1 tablespoon drippings from skillet; heat over medium heat. Add onion; cook and stir 5 minutes or until onion is softened. Add jalapeño and garlic; cook and stir 30 seconds. Remove from heat. Place onion mixture and all but ¼ cup bacon in crust; sprinkle with ¾ cup Cheddar cheese.

3 Whisk eggs, milk and ¼ teaspoon salt in large bowl until well blended. Pour into crust.

4 Bake 30 minutes. Sprinkle with remaining ¼ cup Cheddar cheese and remaining ¼ cup bacon; bake 5 minutes or until cheese is melted. Cut into six squares to serve.

Nutrients Per Serving (1 square)

CALORIES 470 **TOTAL FAT** 36g **CARBS** 10g **NET CARBS** 8g
DIETARY FIBER 2g **PROTEIN** 27g

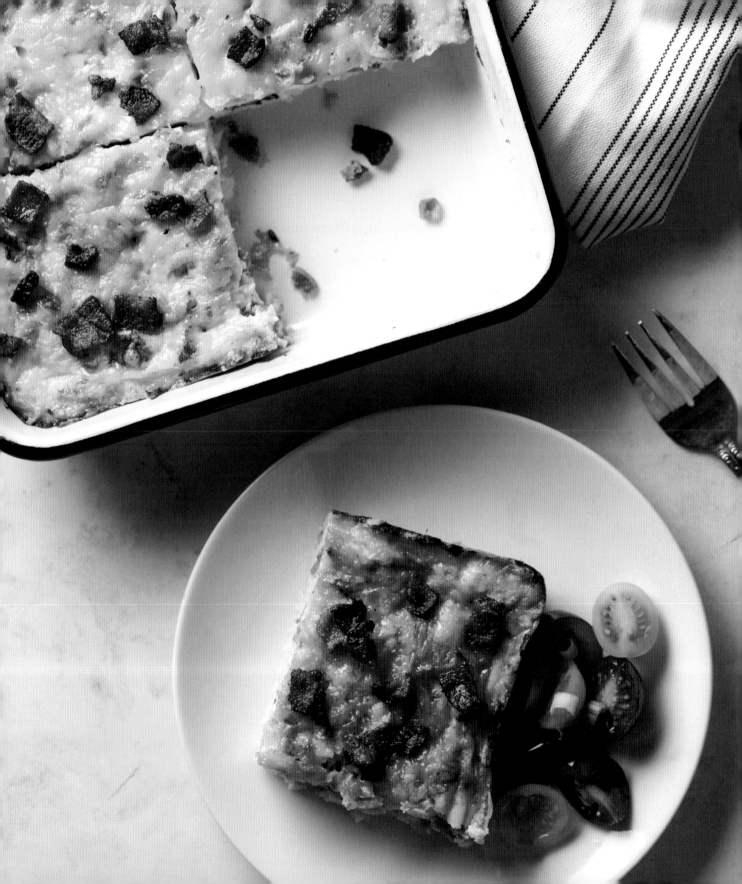

1 container (8 ounces) whipped cream cheese

4 ounces smoked salmon, finely chopped

½ cup finely chopped tomatoes

¼ cup minced green onions

2 teaspoons capers, drained

Sliced Everything Bagels (page 12), cut up bell peppers or keto-friendly crackers

Smoked Salmon Spread

MAKES 1¾ CUPS (ABOUT 12 SERVINGS)

1 Combine cream cheese, salmon, tomatoes, green onions and capers in medium bowl; mix well.

2 Serve with bagels, bell peppers or crackers. Store leftovers in the refrigerator.

Note: Don't use top-quality smoked salmon in this recipe; less expensive salmon works well.

Nutrients Per Serving (2 tablespoons dip)

CALORIES 80   TOTAL FAT 7g   CARBS 2g   NET CARBS 2g
DIETARY FIBER 0g   PROTEIN 3g

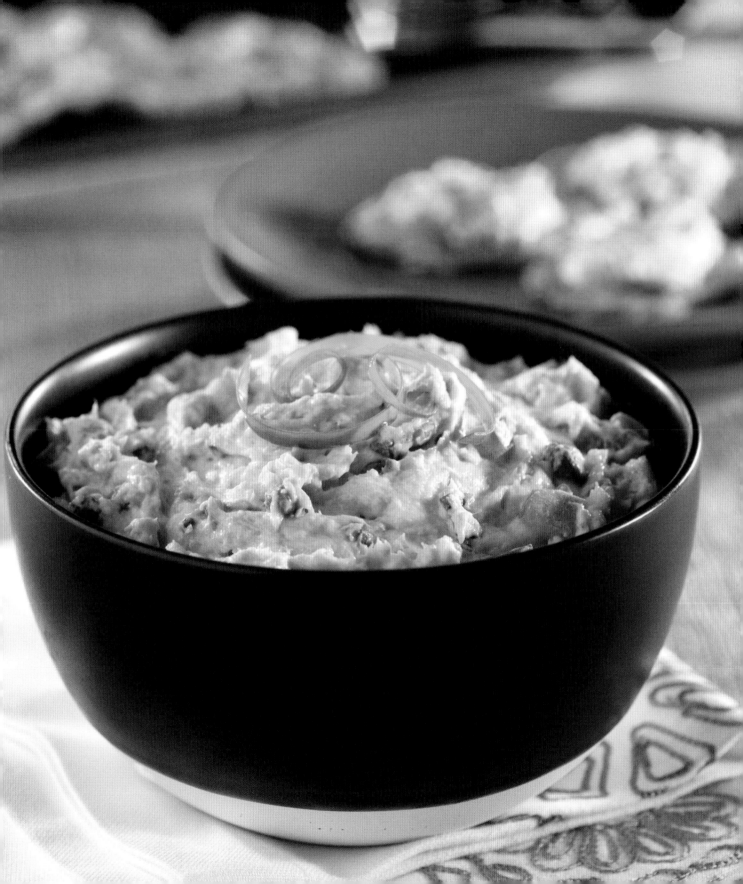

7 tablespoons butter, divided

2 cups almond flour

3½ teaspoons baking powder

½ teaspoon salt

6 eggs at room temperature, separated*

¼ teaspoon cream of tartar

Discard 1 egg yolk.

Keto Bread

MAKES 1 LOAF (16 SLICES)

1 Preheat oven to 375°F. Generously grease 8×4-inch loaf pan with 1 tablespoon butter. Melt remaining 6 tablespoons butter; cool slightly.

2 Combine almond flour, baking powder and salt in medium bowl. Add melted butter and 5 egg yolks; stir until blended.

3 Place egg whites and cream of tartar in bowl of electric stand mixer; attach whip attachment to mixer. Whip egg whites on high speed 1 to 2 minutes or until stiff peaks form.

4 Stir one third of egg whites into almond flour mixture until well blended (batter will be very stiff). Gently fold in remaining egg whites until thoroughly blended (batter may look mottled). Scrape batter into prepared pan; smooth top.

5 Bake 25 to 30 minutes or until top is light brown and dry and toothpick inserted into center comes out clean. Cool in pan on wire rack 10 minutes. Remove from pan; cool completely.

Nutrients Per Serving (1 slice)

CALORIES 156 **TOTAL FAT** 13g **CARBS** 4g **NET CARBS** 2g
DIETARY FIBER 2g **PROTEIN** 5g

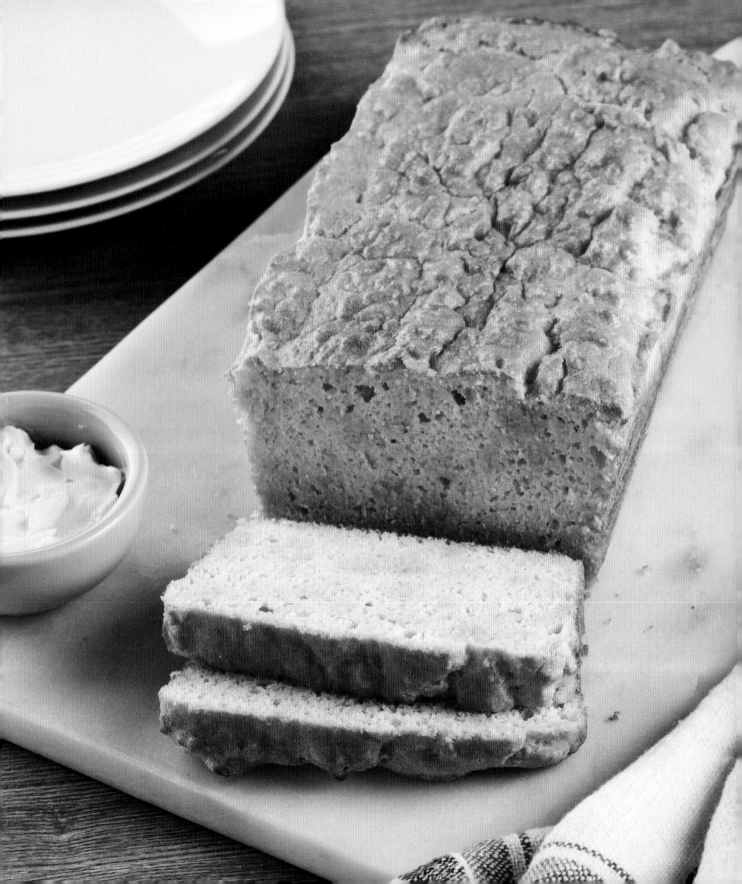

Crust

¾ cup coconut flour

¾ cup almond flour

¼ teaspoon salt

2 eggs

6 tablespoons coconut
  oil or butter, melted

Filling

8 eggs

½ cup whipping cream

1 package (12 ounces)
  bacon

1 cup chopped onion

3 cups tightly packed
  chopped stemmed
  kale

½ cup finely shredded
  Parmesan cheese

¼ cup finely chopped
  sun-dried tomatoes

Bacon-Kale Quiche

MAKES 6 SERVINGS

1 Preheat oven to 375°F. Combine coconut flour, almond
  flour and salt in medium bowl. Stir in 2 eggs and
  coconut oil until well blended. Press onto bottom and
  up side of deep-dish pie plate. Bake 5 minutes.

2 Whisk eggs and cream in large bowl until well blended.
  Cook bacon in large skillet until crisp. Drain on paper
  towels; chop when cool enough to handle. Add onion
  and kale to drippings in skillet; cook and stir over
  medium heat about 5 minutes or until onion is golden
  and kale is wilted. Add vegetables and drippings to
  eggs; mix well. Stir in cheese, tomatoes and bacon.
  Pour into prepared crust.

3 Bake 40 minutes or until quiche is puffed and knife
  inserted into center comes out clean, covering
  edges of crust with foil after 20 minutes to prevent
  overbrowning. Let stand 20 minutes before cutting.

Nutrients Per Serving (1 wedge)

CALORIES 730 **TOTAL FAT** 61g **CARBS** 17g **NET CARBS** 9g
DIETARY FIBER 8g **PROTEIN** 26g

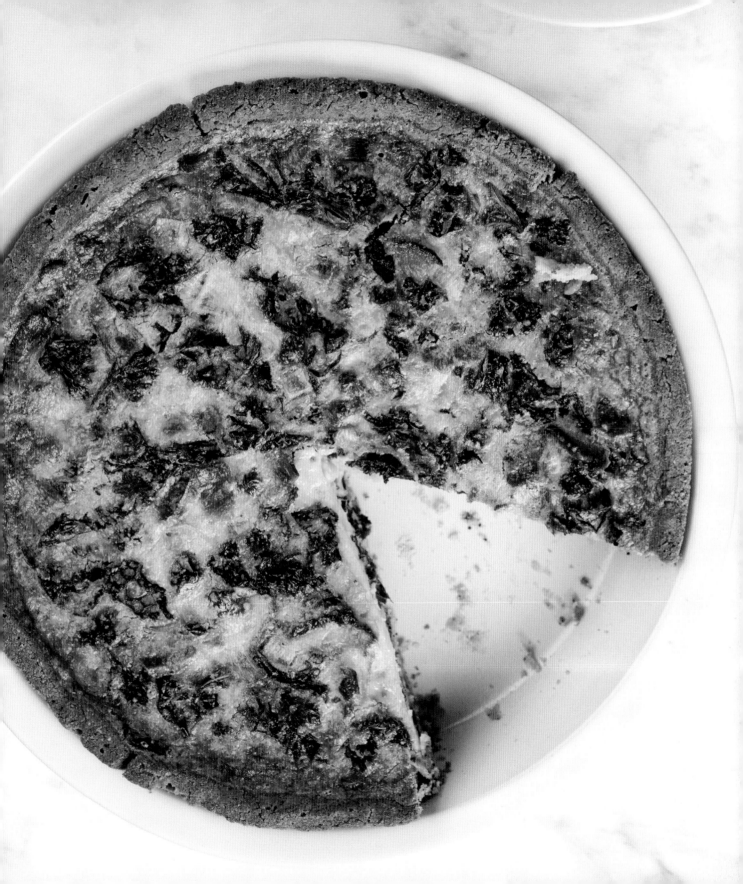

1 tablespoon olive oil

1 small red onion, finely chopped

1½ cups sliced asparagus (½-inch pieces)

1 clove garlic, minced

12 thin slices prosciutto

8 eggs

½ cup (2 ounces) shredded white Cheddar cheese

¼ cup grated Parmesan cheese

2 tablespoons whipping cream

⅛ teaspoon black pepper

Asparagus Frittata Prosciutto Cups
MAKES 12 CUPS

1 Preheat oven to 375°F. Spray 12 standard (2½-inch) muffin cups with nonstick cooking spray.

2 Heat oil in large skillet over medium heat. Add onion; cook and stir 4 minutes or until softened. Add asparagus and garlic; cook and stir 8 minutes or until asparagus is crisp-tender. Set aside to cool slightly.

3 Line each prepared muffin cup with prosciutto slice. (Prosciutto should cover cup as much as possible, with edges extending above muffin pan.) Whisk eggs, Cheddar and Parmesan cheeses, cream and pepper in large bowl until well blended. Stir in asparagus mixture until blended. Pour into prosciutto-lined cups, filling about three-fourths full.

4 Bake about 20 minutes or until frittatas are puffed and golden brown and edges are pulling away from pan. Cool in pan 10 minutes. Remove to wire rack; serve warm or at room temperature.

Nutrients Per Serving (2 frittata cups)

CALORIES 270   TOTAL FAT 18g   CARBS 5g   NET CARBS 4g
DIETARY FIBER 1g   PROTEIN 22g

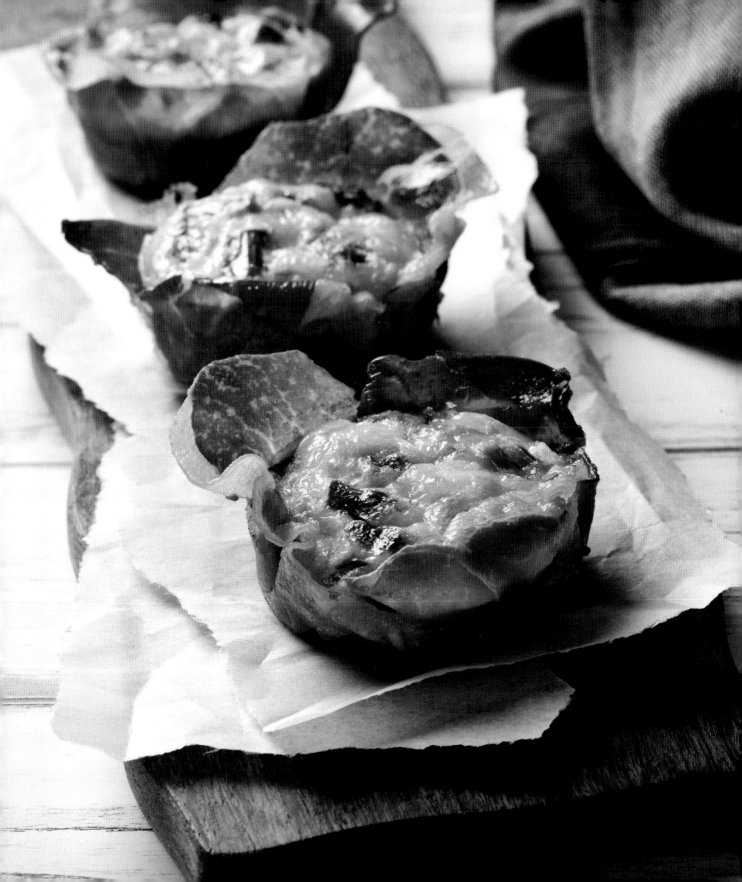

1 pint grape tomatoes

1 tablespoon olive oil

Salt and black pepper

2½ cups riced cauliflower (fresh or frozen)

½ cup Parmesan cheese

6 eggs, divided

¾ teaspoon salt, divided

¼ teaspoon black pepper

¾ cup milk

½ cup (2 ounces) shredded mozzarella cheese

2 cloves garlic, minced

½ teaspoon fresh thyme leaves

Roasted Tomato Quiche

MAKES 6 SERVINGS

1 Preheat oven to 350°F. Place tomatoes in shallow baking dish; drizzle with oil and sprinkle lightly with salt and pepper. Bake 1 hour, stirring once or twice.

2 Spray 9-inch pie plate with nonstick cooking spray. Place cauliflower in large microwavable bowl; cover with plastic wrap and cut slit to vent. Microwave on HIGH 4 minutes; stir. Cover and cook on HIGH 4 minutes. Remove cover; cool slightly. Place cauliflower on double layer of paper towels; fold over paper towels and squeeze to remove excess moisture. Return to bowl. Add Parmesan cheese, 1 egg, ½ teaspoon salt and ¼ teaspoon pepper; mix well. Press onto bottom and up side of prepared pie plate. *Increase oven temperature to 425°F.* Bake crust 15 minutes. Remove from oven; place on sheet pan.

3 *Reduce oven temperature to 375°F.* Whisk remaining 5 eggs, milk, mozzarella cheese, garlic, thyme, ¼ teaspoon salt and a dash of black pepper in medium bowl until well blended. Place tomatoes in crust; pour egg mixture over tomatoes.

4 Bake 45 minutes or until thin knife inserted into center comes out clean (a little cheese is okay). Cool 10 minutes before slicing.

Nutrients Per Serving (1 wedge)

CALORIES 190   **TOTAL FAT** 12g   **CARBS** 8g   **NET CARBS** 7g
DIETARY FIBER 1g   **PROTEIN** 14g

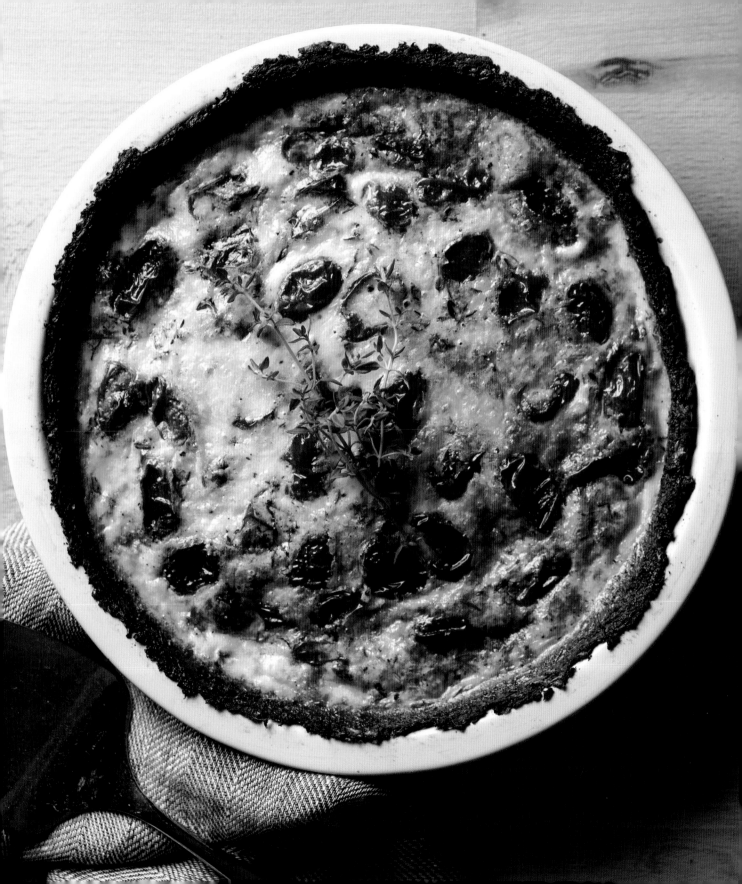

1 cup (8 ounces) hot
   brewed coffee

1 tablespoon butter

1 tablespoon coconut
   oil or MCT oil

1 tablespoon whipping
   cream

Keto Coffee

MAKES 1 SERVING

1 Combine all ingredients in blender container; blend until frothy. Or combine all ingredients in medium bowl and whisk until well blended and frothy.

2 Serve immediately.

Nutrients Per Serving (1 cup)

CALORIES 280   **TOTAL FAT** 300g   **CARBS** 0g   **NET CARBS** 0g
DIETARY FIBER 0g   **PROTEIN** 1g

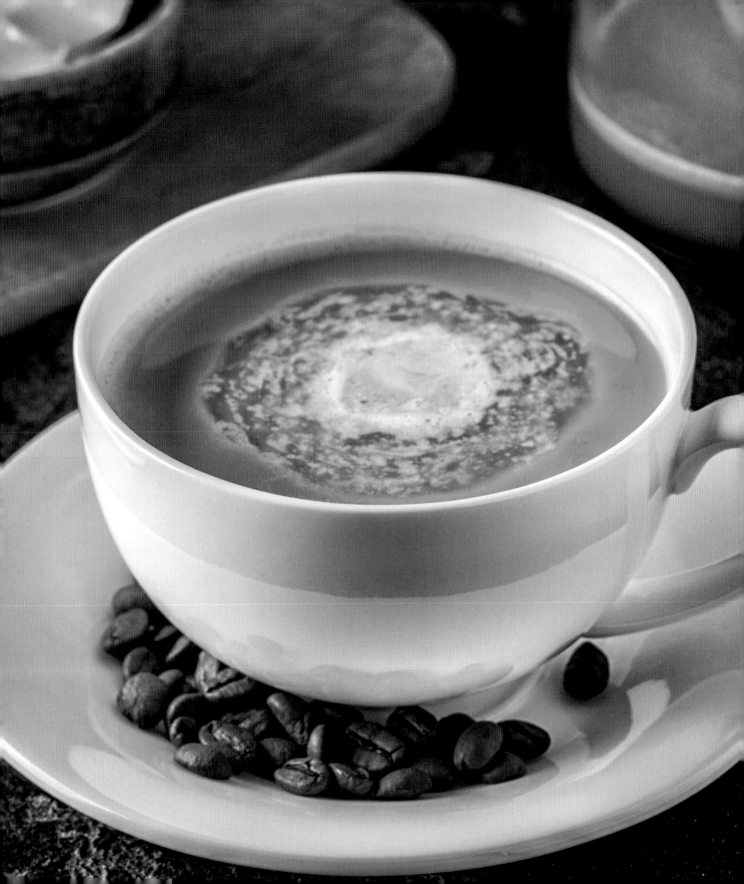

4 eggs

2 cups (8 ounces) shredded Cheddar cheese

½ cup almond flour

½ cup shredded Parmesan cheese

Cheese Waffles

MAKES 4 SERVINGS

1 Preheat waffle iron on medium-high heat.

2 For each waffle, combine 1 egg, ½ cup Cheddar cheese, 2 tablespoons almond flour and 2 tablespoons Parmesan cheese in small bowl until well blended. Pour into hot waffle iron; cook 2 minutes or until waffle is golden brown and releases easily from waffle iron. Place on plate; let stand 2 minutes. Repeat with remaining ingredients to make four waffles.

Nutrients Per Serving (1 waffle)

CALORIES 350   **TOTAL FAT** 27g   **CARBS** 6g   **NET CARBS** 4g
DIETARY FIBER 2g   **PROTEIN** 27g

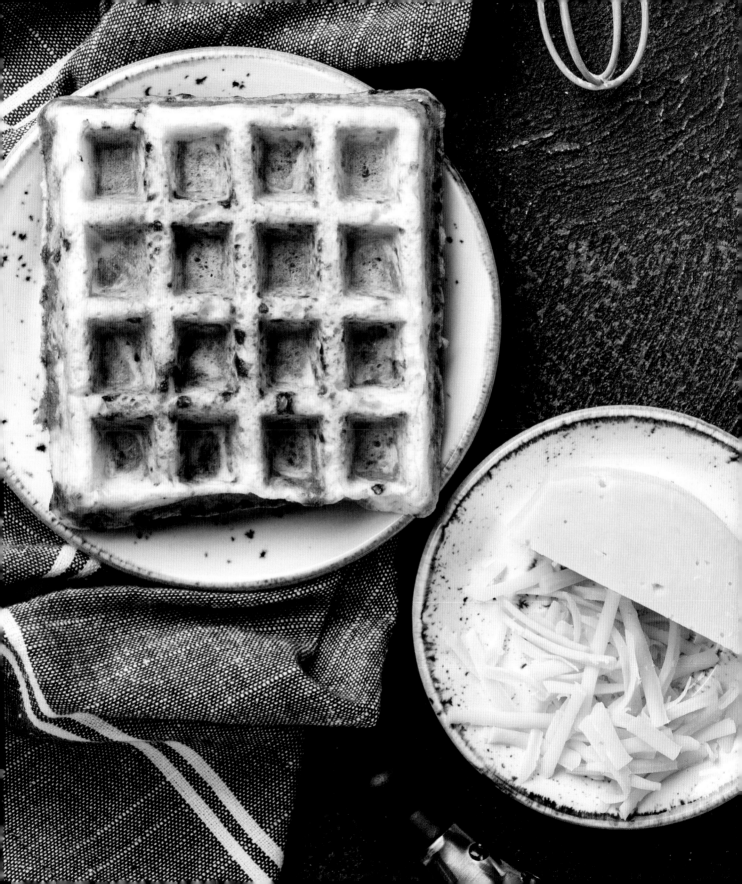

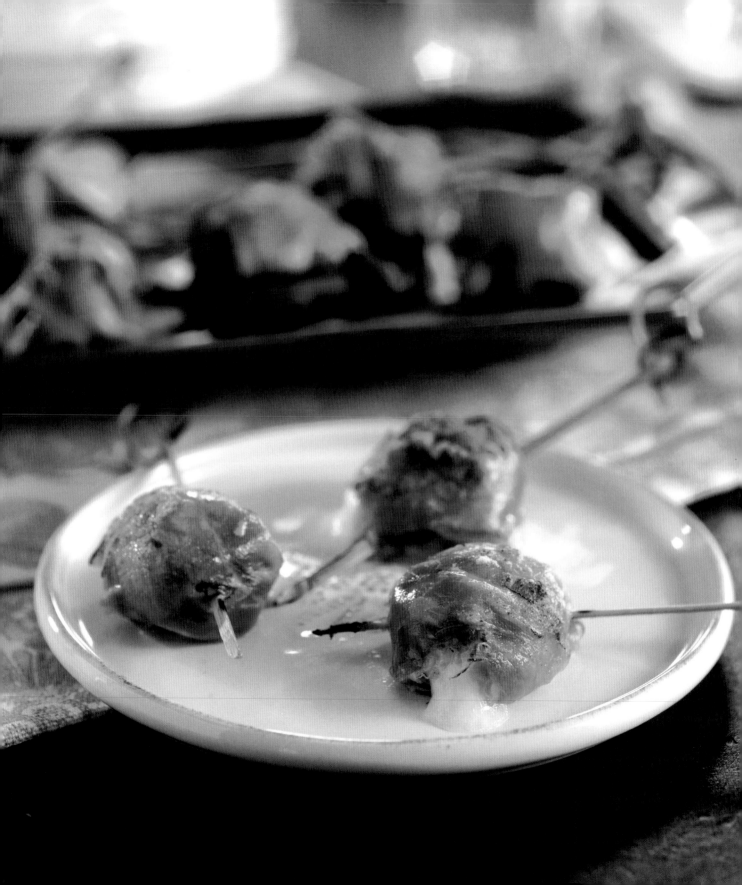

Snacks and Appetizers

Mozzarella and Prosciutto Bites

MAKES 16 TO 20 PIECES

1 Soak skewers in water 20 minutes to prevent burning. Cut mozzarella into 1- to 1½-inch chunks.* Place on paper towel-lined plate; sprinkle with basil and pepper, turning to coat all sides.

2 Cut prosciutto slices crosswise into thirds. Tightly wrap one slice prosciutto around each piece of mozzarella, covering completely. Insert skewer into each piece. Freeze skewers 15 minutes to firm.

3 Preheat broiler. Line broiler pan or baking sheet with foil. Place skewers on prepared pan; broil about 3 minutes or until prosciutto begins to crisp, turning once. Serve immediately.

You can also substitute one 8-ounce container of small fresh mozzarella balls (ciliengini). One 8-ounce container contains 24 balls.

16 to 20 small bamboo skewers or toothpicks

8 ounces fresh mozzarella

¼ cup chopped fresh basil

½ teaspoon black pepper

6 to 8 thin slices prosciutto

Nutrients Per Serving (1 piece)

CALORIES 50 **TOTAL FAT** 4g **CARBS** 0g **NET CARBS** 0g
DIETARY FIBER 0g **PROTEIN** 4g

2 packages (8 ounces each) cream cheese, softened and cut into pieces

1 jar (12 ounces) keto-friendly wing sauce

1 cup keto ranch dressing

2 cups shredded cooked chicken (from 1 pound boneless skinless chicken breasts)

2 cups (8 ounces) shredded Cheddar cheese

Celery sticks

Buffalo Chicken Dip
MAKES 5 CUPS (20 SERVINGS)

1 Combine cream cheese, wing sauce and ranch dressing in large saucepan; cook over medium-low heat 7 to 10 minutes or until cream cheese is melted and mixture is smooth, whisking frequently.

2 Combine chicken and Cheddar cheese in large bowl. Add cream cheese mixture; stir until well blended. Pour into serving bowl; serve warm with celery sticks.

Nutrients Per Serving (¼ cup)

CALORIES 190   **TOTAL FAT** 15g   **CARBS** 3g   **NET CARBS** 3g
DIETARY FIBER 0g   **PROTEIN** 9g

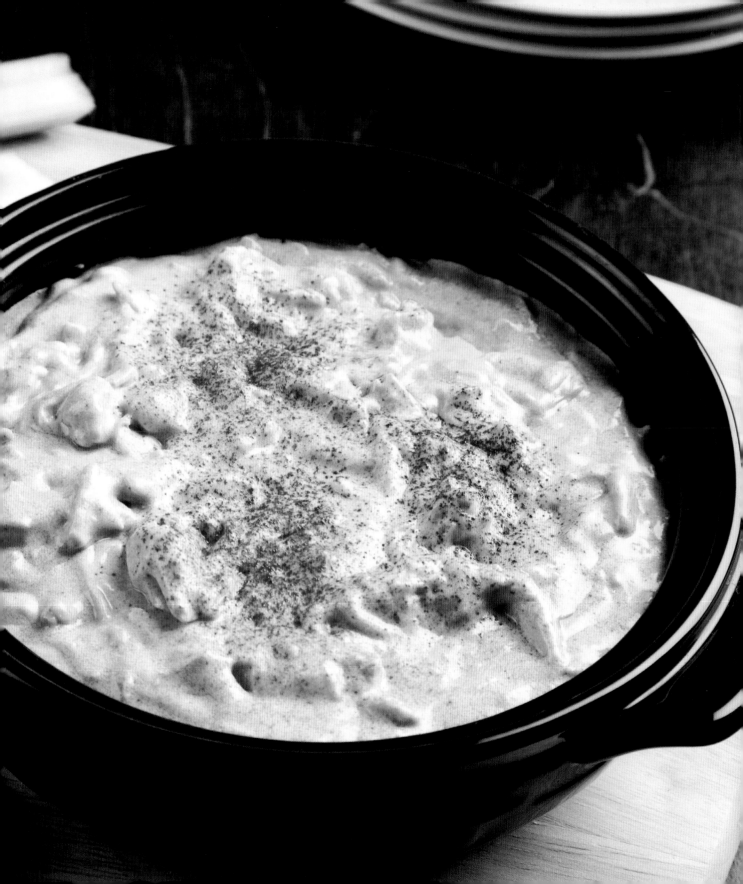

4 eggs

⅛ teaspoon black
pepper

¼ cup chive and onion
cream cheese,
softened

1 package (about
4 ounces) smoked
salmon (lox), cut
into bite-size pieces

Smoked Salmon Omelet Roll-Ups
MAKES ABOUT 24 PIECES (6 SERVINGS)

1 Beat eggs and pepper in small bowl until well blended
(no streaks of white showing). Spray large nonstick
skillet with nonstick cooking spray; heat over medium-
high heat.

2 Pour half of egg mixture into skillet; tilt skillet to
completely coat bottom with thin layer of eggs. Cook,
without stirring, 2 to 4 minutes or until eggs are set.
Use spatula to carefully loosen omelet from skillet; slide
onto cutting board. Repeat with remaining egg mixture
to make second omelet.

3 Spread 2 tablespoons cream cheese over each omelet;
top with smoked salmon pieces. Roll up omelets tightly;
wrap in plastic wrap and refrigerate at least 30 minutes.
Cut off ends, then cut rolls crosswise into ½-inch slices.

Nutrients Per Serving (4 pieces)
CALORIES 100   **TOTAL FAT** 5g   **CARBS** 1g   **NET CARBS** 1g
DIETARY FIBER 0g   **PROTEIN** 14g

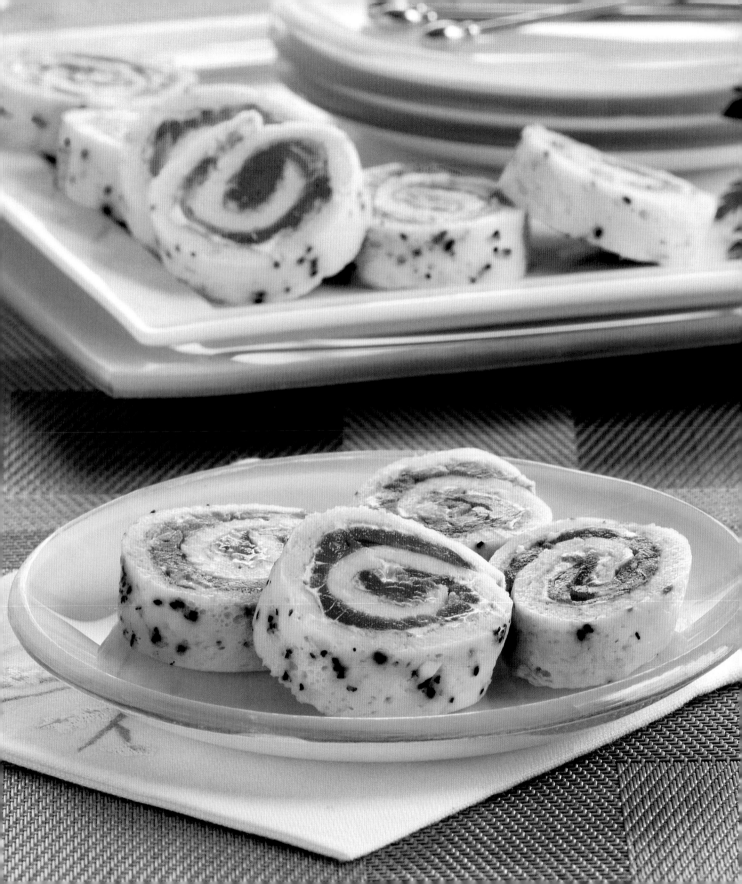

Spicy Chicken Bundles
MAKES 12 APPETIZERS

1 pound ground chicken or turkey

2 teaspoons minced fresh ginger

2 cloves garlic, minced

¼ teaspoon red pepper flakes

1 tablespoon peanut or vegetable oil

3 tablespoons soy sauce

⅓ cup finely chopped water chestnuts

⅓ cup thinly sliced green onions

¼ cup chopped peanuts

12 large lettuce leaves, such as romaine

Chinese hot mustard (optional)

1 Combine chicken, ginger, garlic and red pepper flakes in medium bowl.

2 Heat oil in wok or large skillet over medium-high heat. Add chicken mixture; stir-fry 2 to 3 minutes until chicken is cooked through.

3 Add soy sauce; cook and stir 30 seconds. Add water chestnuts, green onions and peanuts; heat through.*

4 Divide filling evenly among lettuce leaves; roll up and secure with toothpicks. Serve warm or at room temperature. Serve with hot mustard, if desired.

Filling may be made ahead to this point; cover and refrigerate up to 4 hours. Reheat until warm. Proceed as directed in step 4.

Nutrients Per Serving (1 bundle)

CALORIES 90 **TOTAL FAT** 6g **CARBS** 3g **NET CARBS** 2g
DIETARY FIBER 1g **PROTEIN** 8g

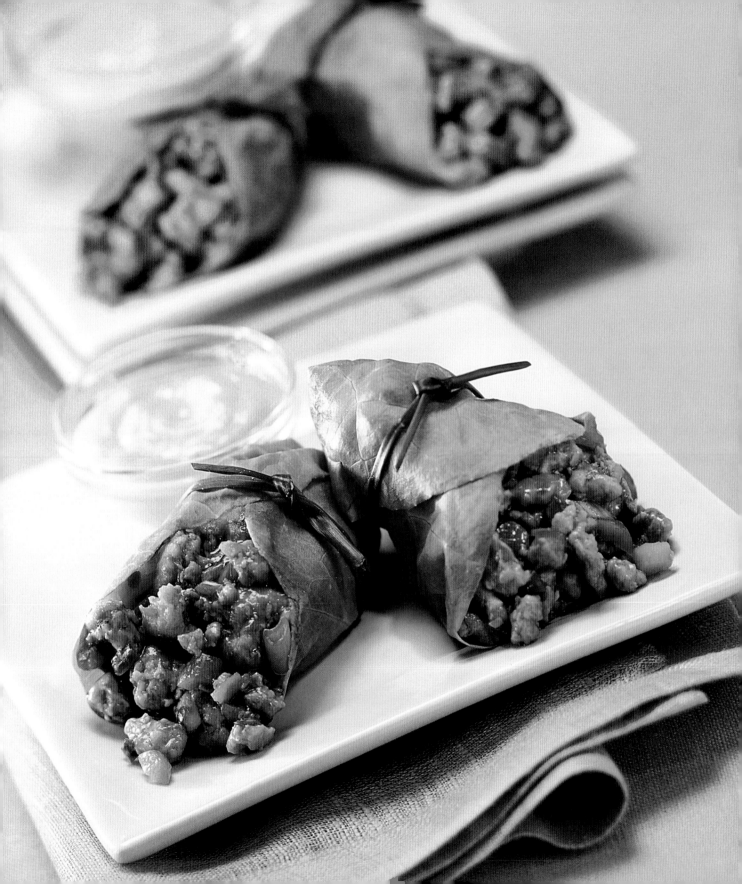

6 eggs

3 tablespoons mayonnaise

½ teaspoon apple cider vinegar

½ teaspoon yellow mustard

⅛ teaspoon salt

Optional toppings: black pepper, paprika, minced fresh chives and/or minced red onion (optional)

Classic Deviled Eggs
MAKES 12 DEVILED EGGS

1 Bring medium saucepan of water to a boil. Gently add eggs with slotted spoon. Reduce heat to maintain a simmer; cook 12 minutes. Meanwhile, fill medium bowl with cold water and ice cubes. Drain eggs and place in ice water; cool 10 minutes.

2 Carefully peel eggs. Cut eggs in half; place yolks in small bowl. Add mayonnaise, vinegar, mustard and salt; mash until well blended. Spoon mixture into egg whites; garnish with desired toppings.

Nutrients Per Serving (1 deviled egg)

CALORIES 30 **TOTAL FAT** 3g **CARBS** 0g **NET CARBS** 0g
DIETARY FIBER 0g **PROTEIN** 2g

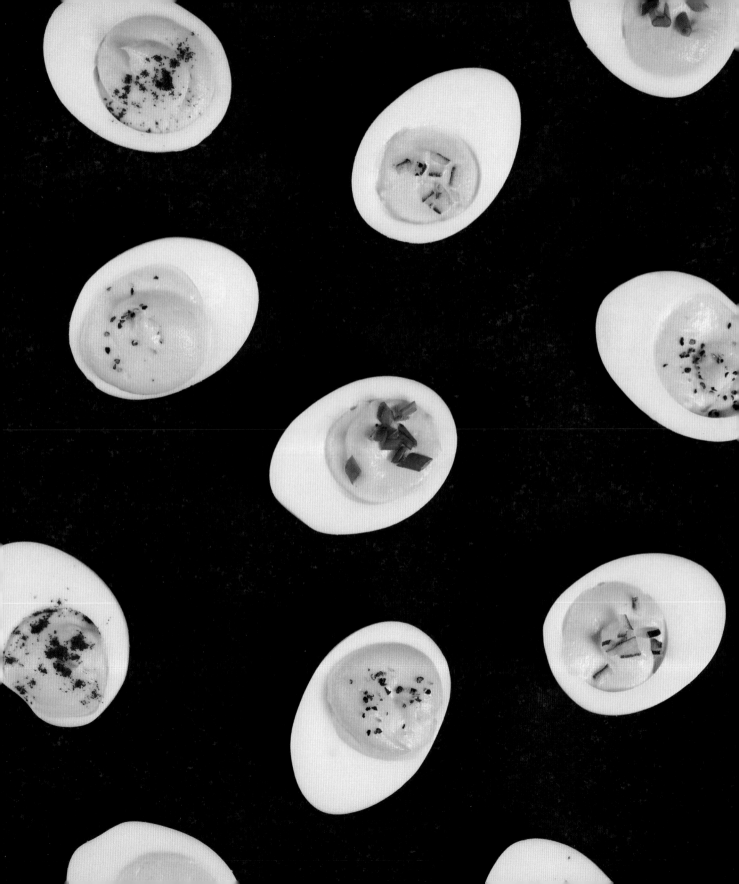

10 to 12 fresh jalapeño peppers*

1 package (8 ounces) cream cheese, softened

1½ cups (6 ounces) shredded Cheddar cheese, divided

2 green onions, finely chopped

½ teaspoon onion powder

¼ teaspoon salt

⅛ teaspoon garlic powder

6 slices bacon, crisp-cooked and finely chopped

2 tablespoons almond flour (optional)

2 tablespoons grated Parmesan or Romano cheese

For large jalapeño peppers, use 10. For small peppers, use 12.

Jalapeño Poppers
MAKES 20 TO 24 POPPERS

1 Preheat oven to 375°F. Line baking sheet with parchment paper or foil.

2 Cut each jalapeño in half lengthwise; remove ribs and seeds.

3 Combine cream cheese, 1 cup Cheddar cheese, green onions, onion powder, salt and garlic powder in medium bowl. Stir in bacon. Fill each jalapeño half with about 1 tablespoon cheese mixture. Place on prepared baking sheet. Sprinkle with remaining ½ cup Cheddar cheese, almond flour, if desired, and Parmesan cheese.

4 Bake 10 to 12 minutes or until cheese is melted but jalapeños are still firm.

Nutrients Per Serving (1 popper)

CALORIES 110 **TOTAL FAT** 10g **CARBS** 2g **NET CARBS** 2g
DIETARY FIBER 0g **PROTEIN** 4g

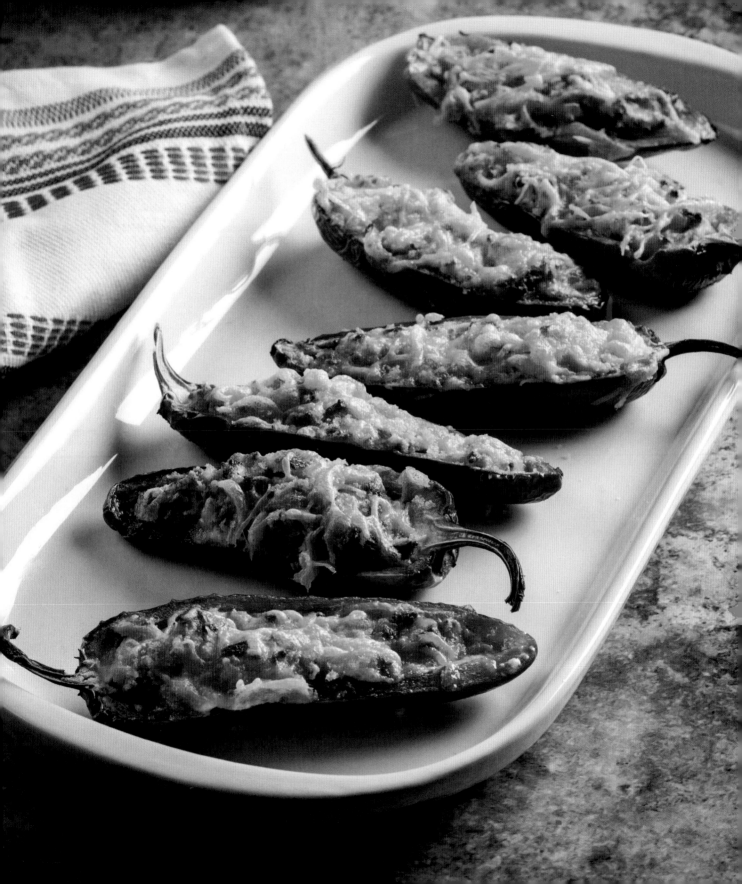

½ (8-ounce) package cream cheese, softened

½ cup sour cream

2 tablespoons mayonnaise

¾ teaspoon seasoned salt

¼ teaspoon paprika, plus additional for garnish

2 cans (6 ounces each) crabmeat, drained and flaked

½ cup (2 ounces) shredded mozzarella cheese

2 tablespoons minced onion

2 tablespoons finely chopped green bell pepper*

Chopped fresh parsley (optional)

For a spicier dip, substitute 1 tablespoon minced jalapeño pepper for the bell pepper.

Crab Dip

MAKES 14 SERVINGS

1 Preheat oven to 350°F.

2 Combine cream cheese, sour cream, mayonnaise, seasoned salt and ¼ teaspoon paprika in medium bowl; stir until well blended and smooth. Add crabmeat, cheese, onion and bell pepper; stir until blended. Spread in small (1-quart) shallow baking dish.

3 Bake 15 to 20 minutes or until bubbly and top is beginning to brown. Garnish with additional paprika and parsley.

Nutrients Per Serving (¼ cup)

CALORIES 110   **TOTAL FAT** 9g   **CARBS** 2g   **NET CARBS** 2g
DIETARY FIBER 0g   **PROTEIN** 6g

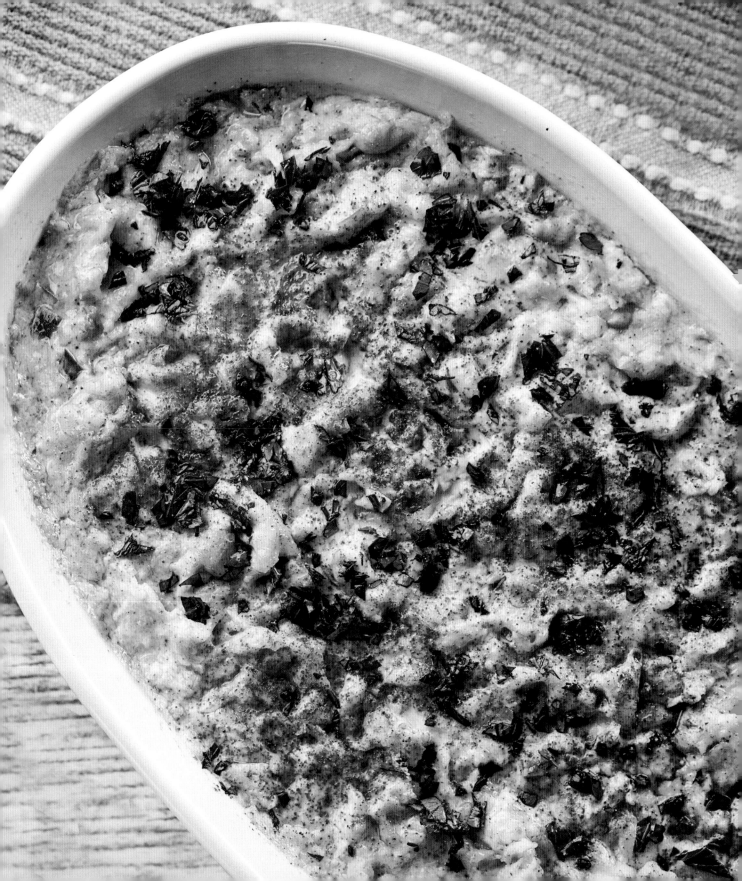

1 pound white mushrooms (about 24 mushrooms), stems removed

2 cans (6 ounces each) lump crabmeat, drained

½ cup (2 ounces) shredded Monterey Jack cheese

⅓ cup finely chopped green onions

3 tablespoons mayonnaise

2 tablespoons shredded Parmesan cheese

1 tablespoon Worcestershire sauce

1 teaspoon minced garlic

2 tablespoons almond flour

Crab Stuffed Mushrooms

MAKES 12 SERVINGS

1 Preheat oven to 350°F. Line baking sheet with parchment paper. Place mushrooms on prepared baking sheet.

2 Combine crabmeat, Monterey Jack cheese, green onions, mayonnaise, Parmesan cheese, Worcestershire sauce and garlic in medium bowl; gently mix. Spoon evenly into mushroom caps, flattening slightly. Sprinkle evenly with almond flour.

3 Bake 20 minutes or until lightly browned.

Nutrients Per Serving (2 stuffed mushrooms)

CALORIES 80 **TOTAL FAT** 6g **CARBS** 2g **NET CARBS** 2g **DIETARY FIBER** 0g **PROTEIN** 3g

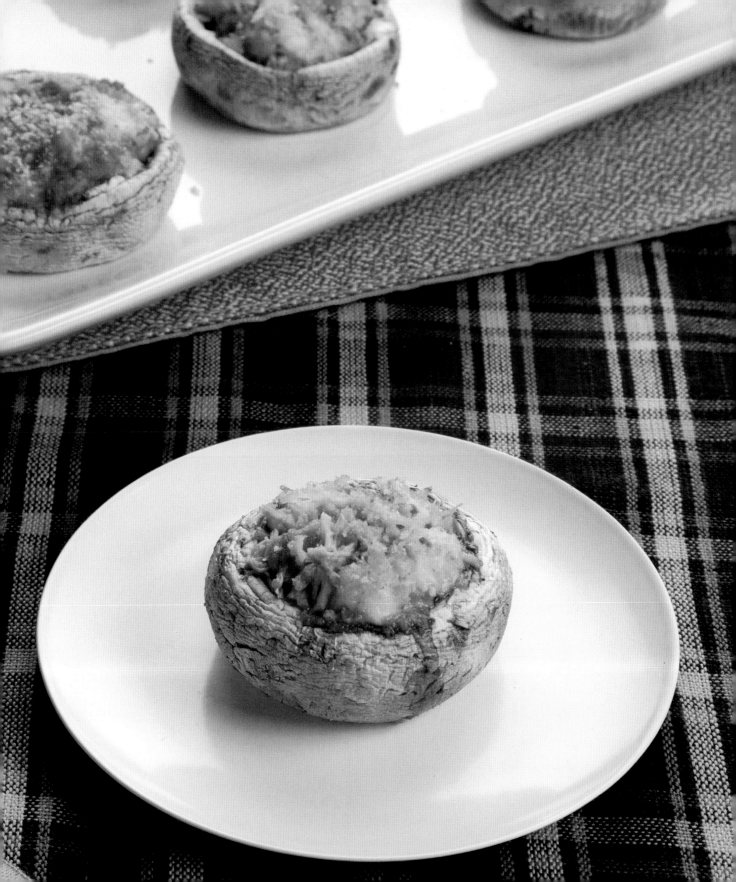

1 cup hot pepper sauce

⅓ cup vegetable oil, plus additional for frying

½ teaspoon ground red pepper

½ teaspoon garlic powder

½ teaspoon Worcestershire sauce

⅛ teaspoon black pepper

1 pound chicken wings, tips discarded, separated at joints

Keto blue cheese or ranch dressing

Celery sticks

Buffalo Wings

MAKES 4 SERVINGS

1 Combine hot pepper sauce, ⅓ cup oil, red pepper, garlic powder, Worcestershire sauce and black pepper in small saucepan; cook over medium heat 20 minutes. Remove from heat; pour sauce into large bowl.

2 Heat 3 inches of oil in large saucepan over medium-high heat to 350°F; adjust heat to maintain temperature. Add wings; cook 10 minutes or until crispy. Drain on wire rack set over paper towels.

3 Transfer wings to bowl of sauce; toss to coat. Serve with blue cheese dressing and celery sticks.

Nutrients Per Serving (¼ pound chicken wings)

CALORIES 320   **TOTAL FAT** 25g   **CARBS** 2g   **NET CARBS** 1g
DIETARY FIBER 1g   **PROTEIN** 20g

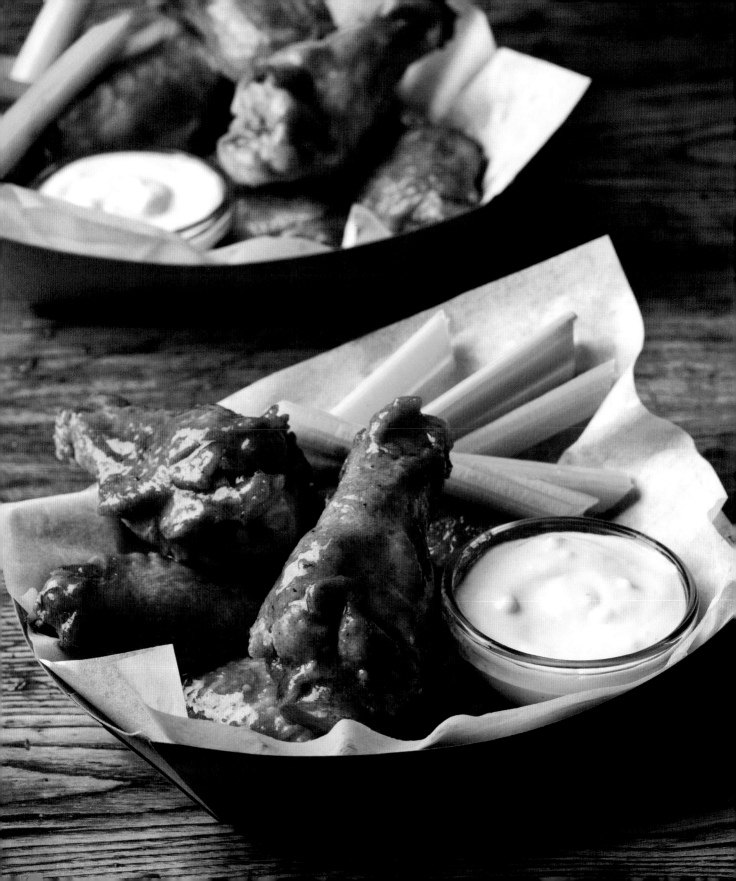

1 medium head
   cauliflower, finely
   chopped and
   squeezed dry
1 cup (4 ounces)
   shredded
   mozzarella cheese
1 cup shredded
   Parmesan cheese,
   divided
¾ cup almond flour
2 cloves garlic, minced
½ teaspoon Italian
   seasoning
1 teaspoon salt
1 egg

Garlic "Bread" Sticks
MAKES 14 STICKS

1 Preheat oven to 425°F. Line sheet pan with parchment
   paper or grease with 1 tablespoon vegetable oil.

2 Combine cauliflower, mozzarella cheese, ½ cup
   Parmesan cheese, almond flour, garlic, Italian seasoning,
   salt and egg in large bowl; mix well. Pat into 12×10-inch
   rectangle on prepared sheet pan.

3 Bake 30 minutes or until well browned and edges
   are crispy. Sprinkle with additional ½ cup shredded
   Parmesan cheese. Bake 10 minutes or until cheese
   is melted. Cut crosswise into 7 strips; cut in half
   lengthwise to make 14 sticks.

Nutrients Per Serving (1 stick)
CALORIES 110   **TOTAL FAT** 8g   **CARBS** 4g   **NET CARBS** 3g
DIETARY FIBER 1g   **PROTEIN** 8g

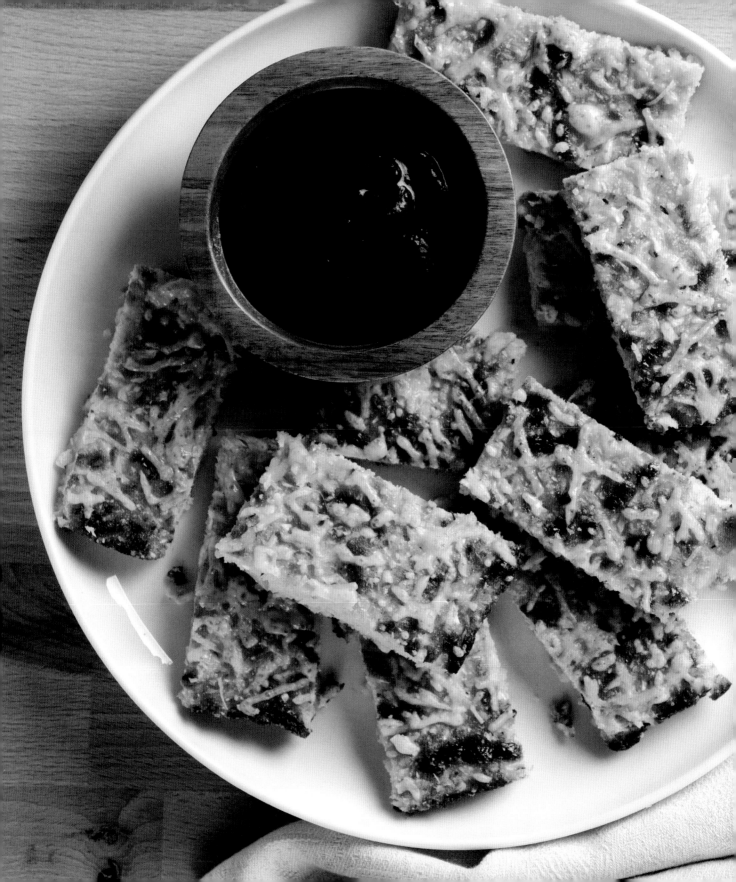

2½ teaspoons salt,
    divided

1 head cauliflower, cut
    into 1-inch florets

½ clove garlic

¾ cup tahini

2 tablespoons lemon
    juice

Olive oil and paprika
    for serving

Sliced raw fennel and/
    or bell pepper strips
    for dipping

Cauliflower Hummus

MAKES 3 CUPS (12 SERVINGS)

1 Fill large saucepan with 1 inch water. Bring to a simmer over medium-high heat; stir in 2 teaspoons salt. Add cauliflower; reduce heat to medium. Cover and cook about 10 minutes or until cauliflower is very tender. Drain and cool slightly.

2 Process cauliflower, garlic and remaining ½ teaspoon salt in food processor 1 minute. Scrape side of bowl. With motor running, add tahini and lemon juice; process 2 minutes or until very smooth and fluffy. Transfer hummus to bowl; drizzle with oil and sprinkle with paprika, if desired. Serve with vegetables.

Nutrients Per Serving (¼ cup)

CALORIES 100   **TOTAL FAT** 7g   **CARBS** 7g   **NET CARBS** 4g
DIETARY FIBER 3g   **PROTEIN** 4g

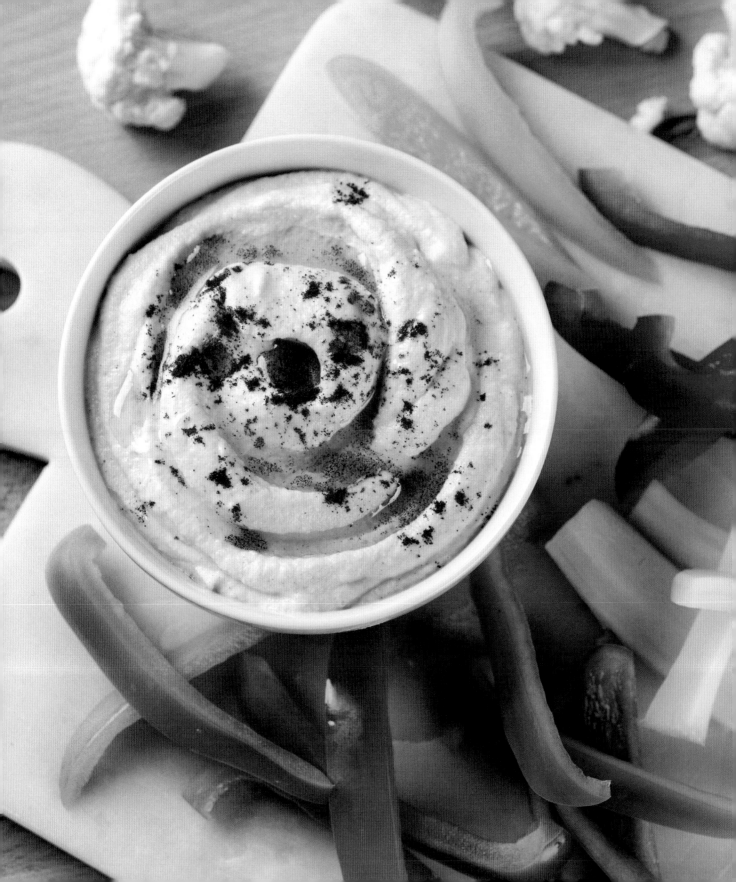

6 tablespoons almond flour

¼ cup grated Parmesan cheese

1 egg white

1 tablespoon water

2 small zucchini (about 4 ounces each), cut lengthwise into quarters

⅓ cup pasta sauce, warmed

Savory Zucchini Sticks
MAKES 4 SERVINGS

1 Preheat oven to 400°F. Spray baking sheet with nonstick cooking spray.

2 Combine almond flour and cheese in shallow dish. Combine egg white and water in another shallow dish; beat with fork until well blended.

3 Dip each piece of zucchini into egg white mixture, letting excess drip back into dish. Roll in cheese mixture to coat. Place zucchini sticks on prepared baking sheet; spray with cooking spray.

4 Bake 15 to 18 minutes or until golden brown. Serve with pasta sauce.

Nutrients Per Serving (2 sticks and 1 tablespoon sauce)
CALORIES 120 **TOTAL FAT** 8g **CARBS** 6g **NET CARBS** 4g
DIETARY FIBER 2g **PROTEIN** 7g

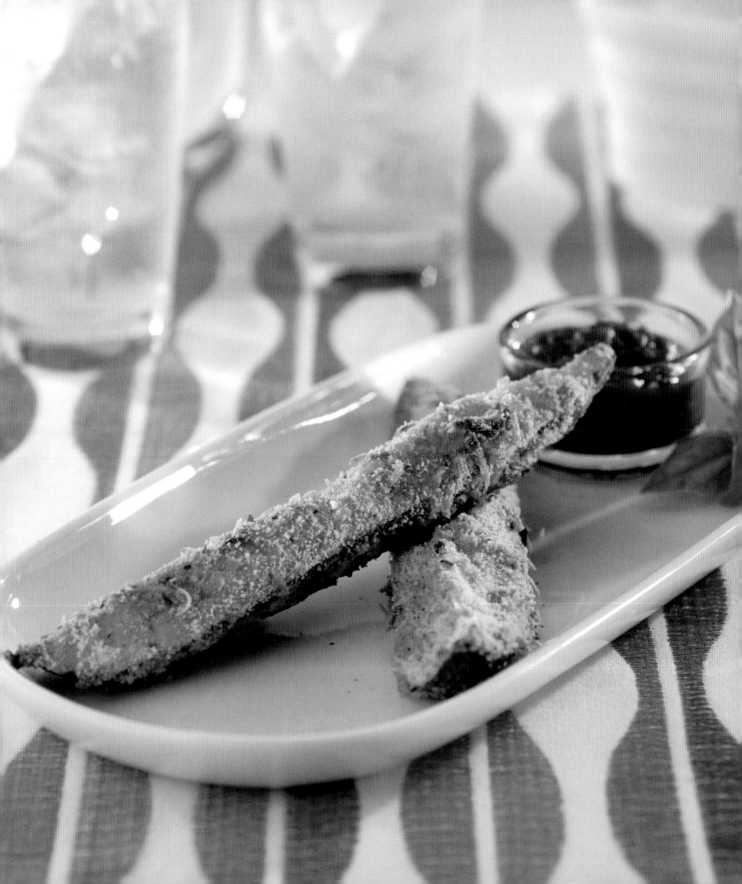

12 ounces cream cheese, softened

½ cup sour cream

2 teaspoons chili powder

1½ teaspoons ground cumin

⅛ teaspoon ground red pepper

½ cup salsa

1 cup (4 ounces) shredded Cheddar cheese

1 cup (4 ounces) shredded Monterey Jack cheese

½ cup diced plum tomatoes

⅓ cup sliced green onions

¼ cup sliced pitted black olives

¼ cup sliced pimiento-stuffed green olives

Shredded lettuce

Keto crackers or cut-up vegetables

Taco Dip

MAKES 10 SERVINGS

1 Combine cream cheese, sour cream, chili powder, cumin and red pepper in large bowl; mix until well blended. Stir in salsa.

2 Spread dip onto serving platter. Top with cheeses, tomatoes, green onions and olives. Sprinkle shredded lettuce around edges of dip.

3 Serve with crackers or vegetables.

Nutrients Per Serving (¹⁄₁₀ of total recipe)

CALORIES 210   **TOTAL FAT** 19g   **CARBS** 5g   **NET CARBS** 4g
DIETARY FIBER 1g   **PROTEIN** 9g

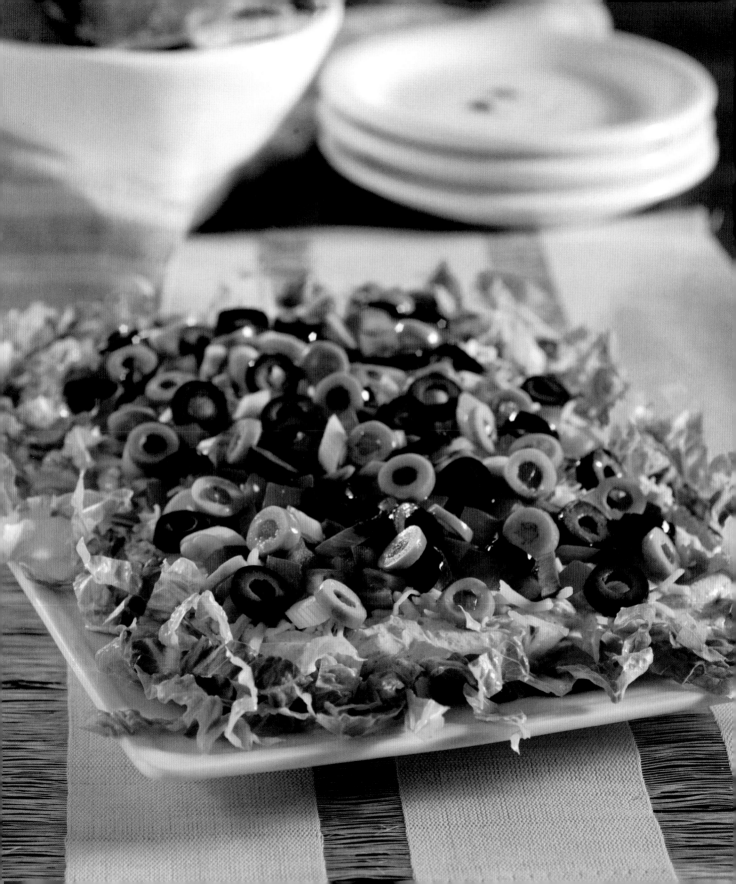

Tirokafteri
(Spicy Greek Feta Spread)
MAKES 2 CUPS

2 small hot red peppers
½ small clove garlic
1 block (8 ounces) feta cheese
¾ cup plain Greek yogurt
1 tablespoon lemon juice
½ teaspoon salt
   Cut-up fresh vegetables

1 Preheat oven to 400°F. Place peppers on small piece of foil or baking sheet. Bake 15 minutes or until peppers are soft and charred. Cool completely. Scrape off skin with paring knife. Cut off top and remove seeds. Place peppers in food processor. Add garlic; pulse until finely chopped.

2 Add feta, yogurt, lemon juice and salt; pulse until well blended but still chunky. Store in airtight jar in refrigerator up to 2 weeks. Serve with vegetables or cooked meats.

Nutrients Per Serving (2 tablespoons)
CALORIES 45 **TOTAL FAT** 3g **CARBS** 1g **NET CARBS** 1g
DIETARY FIBER 0g **PROTEIN** g

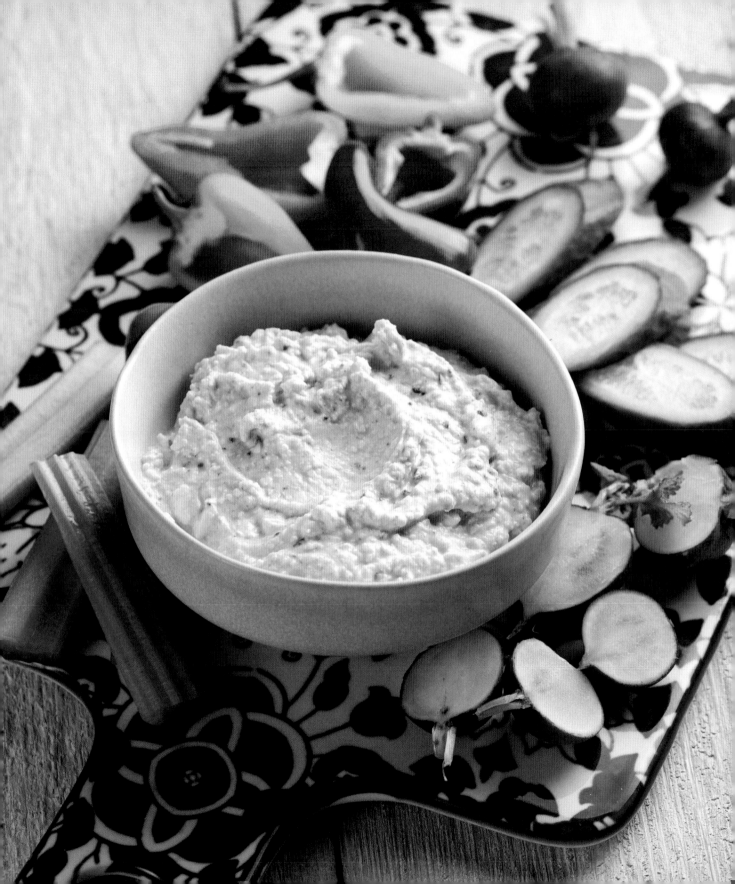

2 packages (8 ounces each) whole mushrooms

1 tablespoon butter

⅔ cup finely chopped cooked chicken

1 tablespoon chopped fresh basil

2 teaspoons lemon juice

⅛ teaspoon onion powder

⅛ teaspoon salt

Pinch garlic powder

Pinch black pepper

¼ cup grated Parmesan cheese

3 ounces cream cheese, softened

Paprika

Stuffed Mushroom Caps

MAKES 24 MUSHROOMS

1 Preheat oven to 350°F. Remove stems from mushrooms and finely chop. Arrange mushroom caps top sides down on greased baking sheet.

2 Melt butter in medium skillet over medium-high heat. Add mushrooms; cook and stir 5 minutes. Add chicken, basil, lemon juice, onion powder, salt, garlic powder and pepper; cook and stir 5 minutes. Remove from heat; stir in Parmesan cheese and cream cheese.

3 Spoon mixture into each mushroom cap. Bake 10 to 15 minutes or until heated through. Sprinkle with paprika.

Nutrients Per Serving (6 mushrooms)

CALORIES 180   **TOTAL FAT** 12g   **CARBS** 5g   **NET CARBS** 4g
DIETARY FIBER 1g   **PROTEIN** 13g

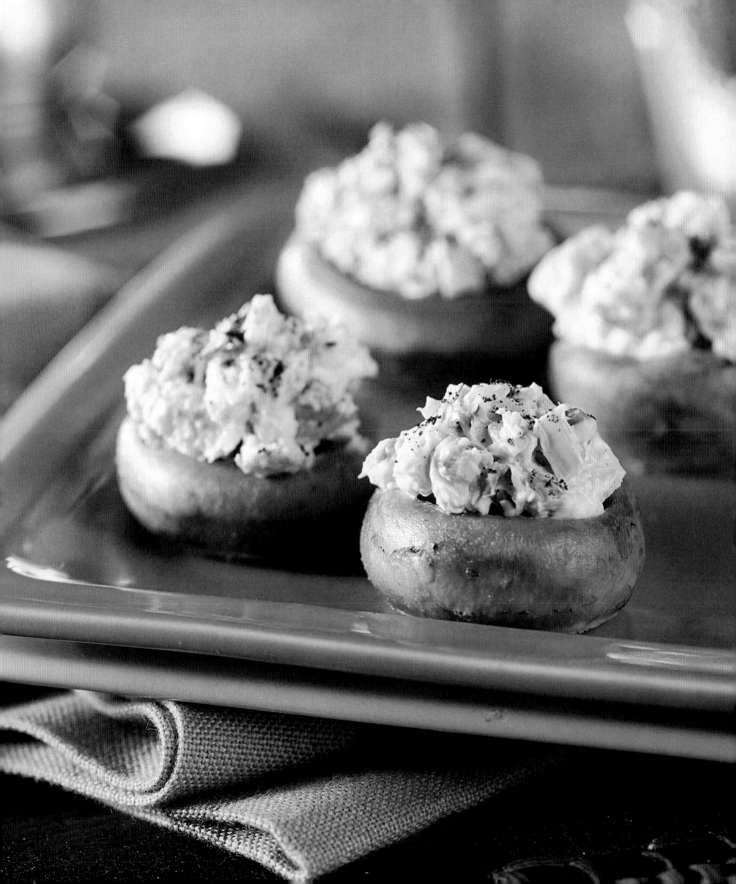

1 cup whole blanched
   almonds
¾ teaspoon olive oil
¼ teaspoon coarse salt
¼ teaspoon smoked
   paprika or paprika

Paprika-Spiced Almonds

MAKES 1 CUP (8 SERVINGS)

1 Preheat oven to 375°F. Spread almonds in single layer in shallow baking pan. Bake 8 to 10 minutes or until almonds are lightly browned. Transfer to bowl; cool 5 to 10 minutes.

2 Toss almonds with oil until completely coated. Sprinkle with salt and paprika; toss again.

Tip: For the best flavor, serve these almonds the day they are made.

Nutrients Per Serving (2 tablespoons)

CALORIES 110   **TOTAL FAT** 10g   **CARBS** 4g   **NET CARBS** 2g
DIETARY FIBER 2g   **PROTEIN** 4g

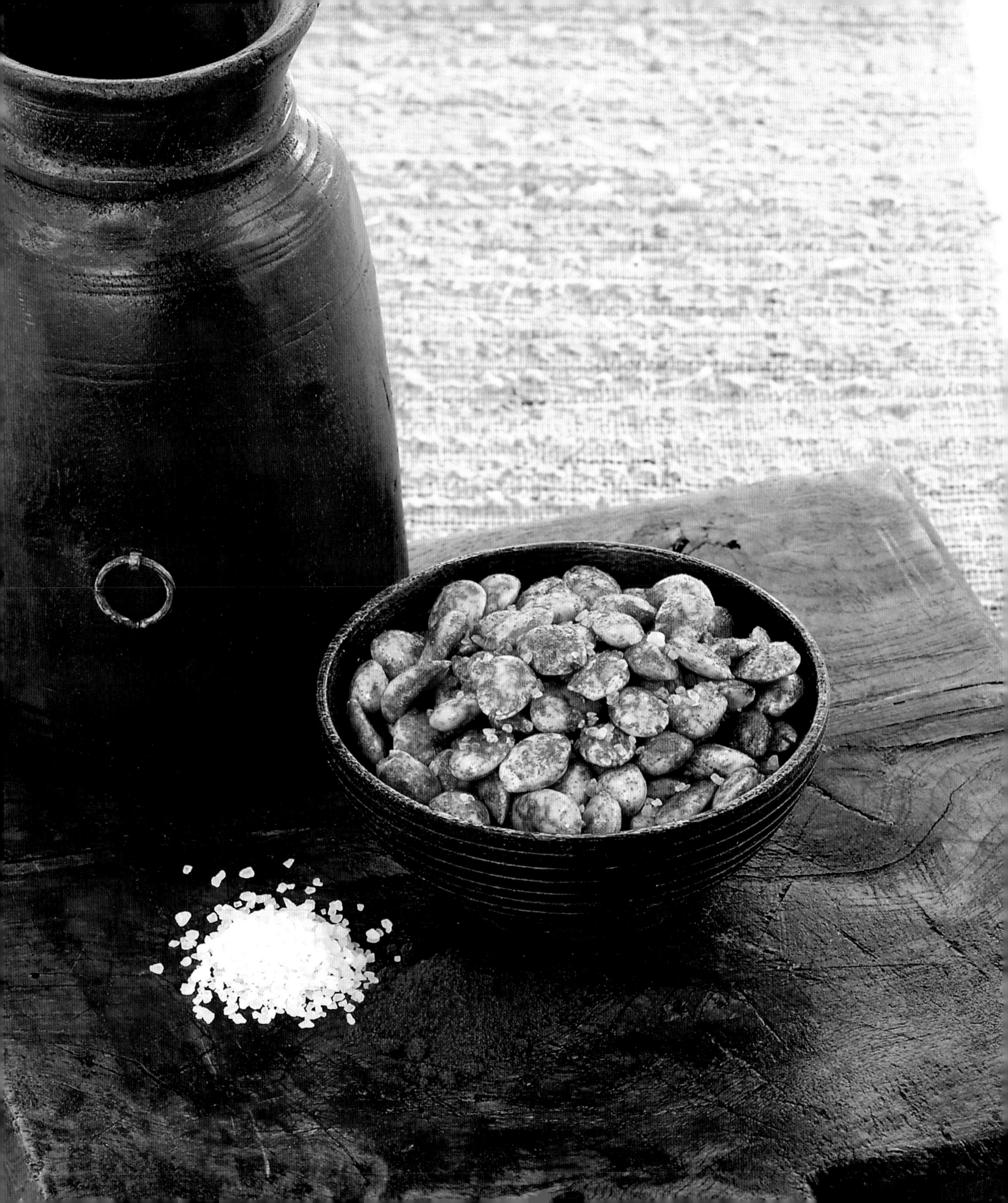

1 to 2 red or yellow bell
    peppers, cut into
    bite-size pieces

16 jumbo sea scallops
    (about 1 pound)

2 tablespoons prepared
    pesto

Pesto Scallop Skewers

MAKES 16 SKEWERS

1 Thread 2 bell pepper pieces and 1 scallop onto each of
16 short wooden skewers. Brush pesto over bell peppers
and scallops.

2 Heat nonstick grill pan or large nonstick skillet over
medium-high heat. Cook skewers 2 to 3 minutes on
each side or until scallops are opaque in center.

Nutrients Per Serving (4 skewers)

CALORIES 120   **TOTAL FAT** 4g   **CARBS** 7g   **NET CARBS** 6g
DIETARY FIBER 1g   **PROTEIN** 14g

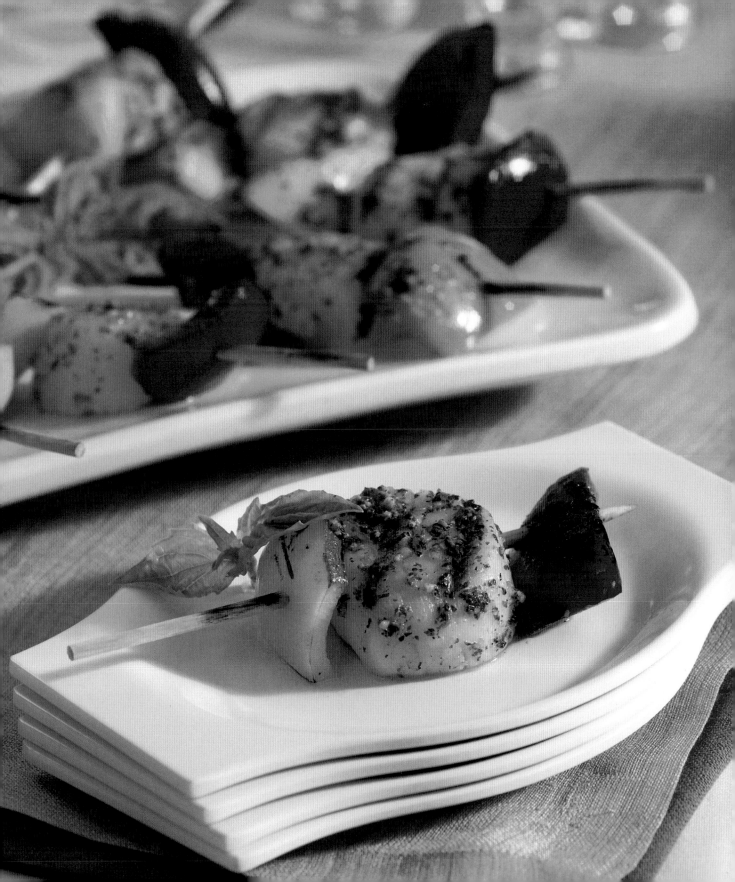

2 tablespoons unsalted butter

2 cups pecan halves

1 cup unsalted macadamia nuts

1 cup walnuts

1 teaspoon dried rosemary

½ teaspoon salt

¼ teaspoon red pepper flakes

Rosemary Nut Mix

MAKES 2 CUPS (32 SERVINGS)

1 Preheat oven to 300°F.

2 Melt butter in large saucepan over low heat. Stir in pecans, macadamia nuts and walnuts. Add rosemary, salt and red pepper flakes; cook and stir about 1 minute. Spread mixture on ungreased baking sheet.

3 Bake 8 to 10 minutes, stirring occasionally. Cool completely on baking sheet on wire rack.

Nutrients Per Serving (2 tablespoons)

CALORIES 108 **TOTAL FAT** 11g **CARBS** 2g **NET CARBS** 1g
DIETARY FIBER 1g **PROTEIN** 2g

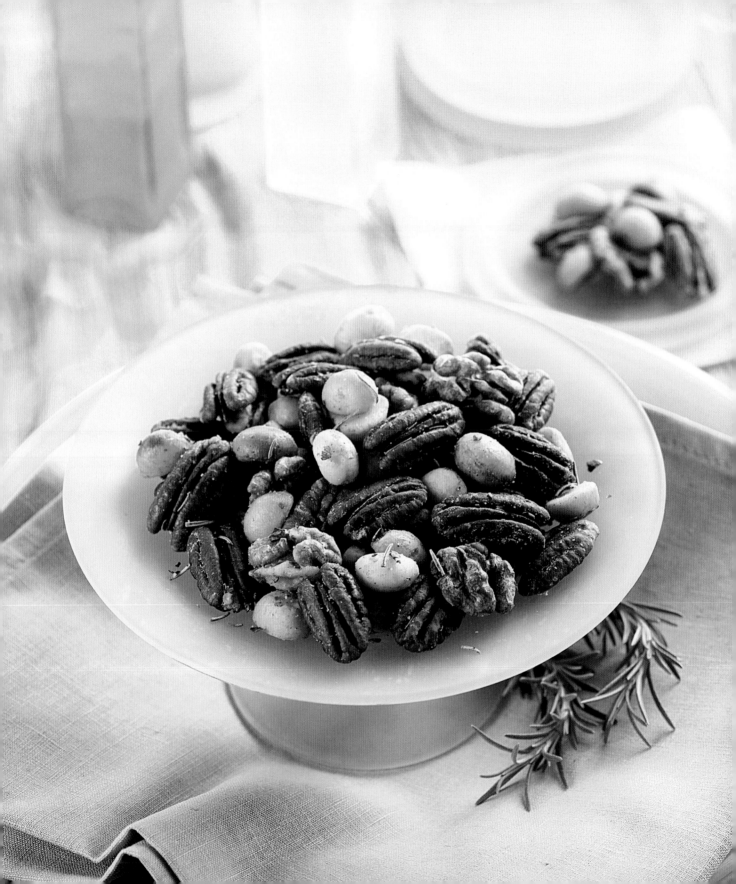

2 ripe avocados

½ cup chunky salsa

¼ teaspoon hot pepper sauce (optional)

½ seedless cucumber, sliced into ⅛-inch-thick rounds

Fast Guacamole

MAKES 8 SERVINGS

1 Cut avocados in half; remove and discard pits. Scoop flesh into medium bowl; mash with fork.

2 Add salsa and hot pepper sauce, if desired; mix well.

3 Transfer guacamole to serving bowl. Serve with cucumber "chips."

Nutrients Per Serving
(3½ tablespoons dip with cucumbers)

CALORIES 156   **TOTAL FAT** 13g   **CARBS** 4g   **NET CARBS** 2g
DIETARY FIBER 2g   **PROTEIN** 5g

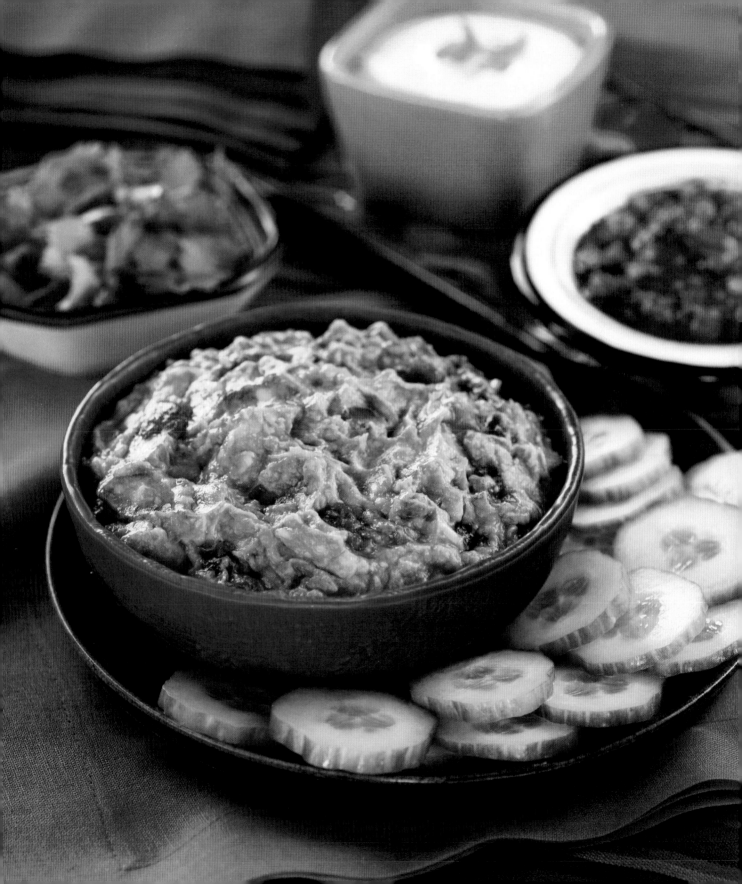

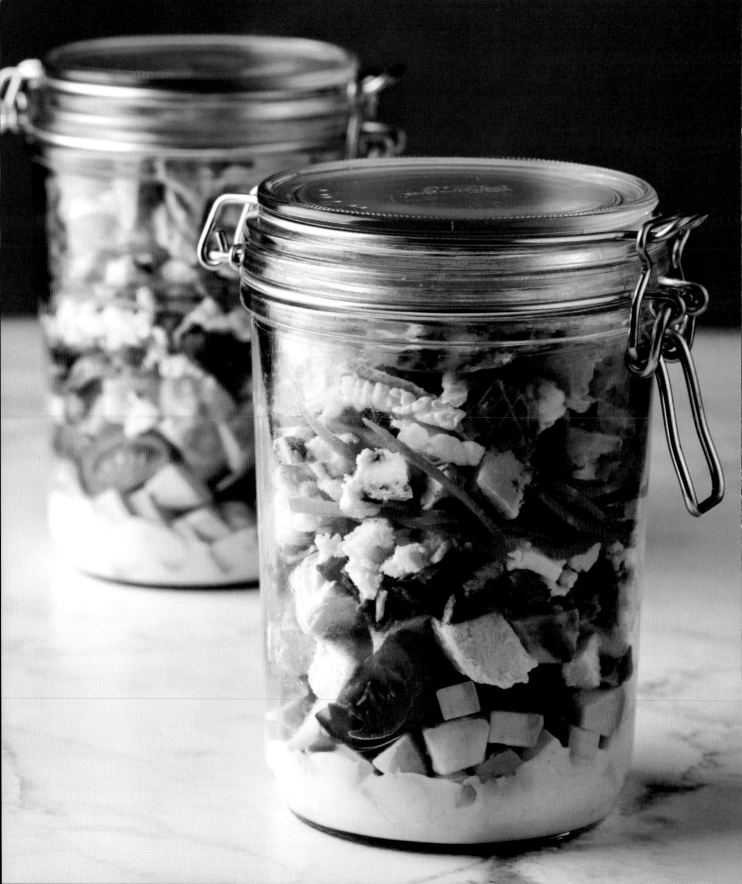

Lunches

Cobb Salad to Go

MAKES 4 SERVINGS

1 Place 2 tablespoons blue cheese dressing into bottom of four (1-quart) jars. Layer remaining ingredients on top, ending with salad greens. Seal jars.

2 Refrigerate until ready to serve.

Nutrients Per Serving (1 jar)

CALORIES 440   **TOTAL FAT** 33g   **CARBS** 12g   **NET CARBS** 6g
DIETARY FIBER 6g   **PROTEIN** 25g

½ cup keto blue cheese dressing

1 ripe avocado, diced

1 tomato, chopped

6 ounces cooked chicken breast, cut into 1-inch pieces

4 slices bacon, crisp-cooked and crumbled

2 hard-cooked eggs, mashed

1 large carrot, shredded

½ cup blue cheese, crumbled

1 package (10 ounces) torn mixed salad greens

Tuna Melt

MAKES 8 SERVINGS

¾ cup mayonnaise

2 teaspoons lemon juice

1 teaspoon salt

⅛ teaspoon black pepper

1 can (12 ounces) solid white albacore tuna, drained

1 can (12 ounces) chunk light tuna, drained

1 stalk celery, finely chopped (about ½ cup)

¼ cup minced red onion

½ loaf Keto Bread (page 20), cut into 8 slices

8 slices Cheddar cheese

2 tablespoons butter

Optional toppings: tomato slices, avocado slices, onion rings, pickles and/or lettuce leaves

1 Combine mayonnaise, lemon juice, salt and pepper in large bowl. Add tuna, celery and onion; mix well.

2 Divide tuna among bread slices; top each with cheese. Heat 1 tablespoon butter in large skillet over medium heat until melted. Add half of sandwiches; cover and cook until bread is toasted and cheese is melted. Repeat with remaining butter and sandwiches. Garnish with desired toppings.

Nutrients Per Serving (1 sandwich)

CALORIES 490 **TOTAL FAT** 40g **CARBS** 4g **NET CARBS** 2g **DIETARY FIBER** 2g **PROTEIN** 31g

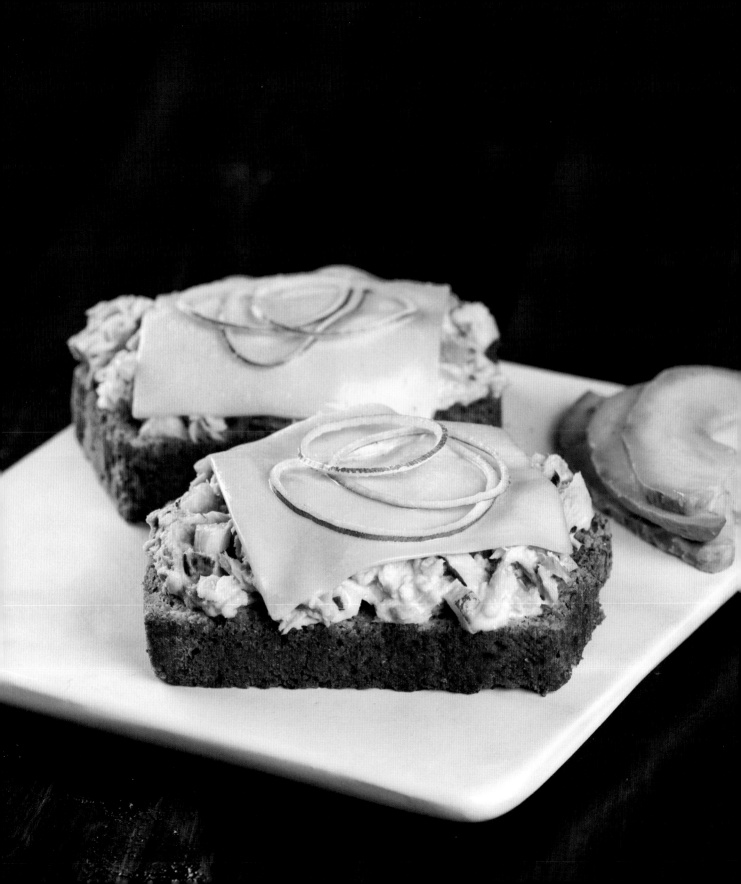

1 boneless pork loin roast (about 3 pounds)

½ cup soy sauce

1 tablespoon chili garlic sauce or chili paste

2 teaspoons minced fresh ginger

2 tablespoons water

1 tablespoon coconut flour

2 teaspoons dark sesame oil

Shredded carrots (optional)

20 large lettuce leaves

Spicy Asian Pork Bundles
MAKES 20 BUNDLES

Slow Cooker Directions

1 Combine pork, soy sauce, chili garlic sauce and ginger in slow cooker; mix well. Cover; cook on LOW 8 to 10 hours.

2 Remove roast to large cutting board; shred with two forks. Turn off heat. Let cooking liquid stand 5 minutes. Skim off and discard fat.

3 Stir water, coconut flour and oil in small bowl until smooth; whisk into cooking liquid. Turn slow cooker to HIGH. Cook, uncovered, on HIGH 10 minutes or until sauce is thickened. Stir in shredded pork. Cover; cook on HIGH 15 to 30 minutes or until heated through.

4 Place ¼ cup pork filling and carrots, if desired, into lettuce leaves. Wrap to enclose. Serve immediately or pack individual servings of pork and lettuce in separate food storage containers to take for lunch.

Nutrients Per Serving (1 bundle)

CALORIES 100 **TOTAL FAT** 4g **CARBS** 1g **NET CARBS** 1g
DIETARY FIBER 0g **PROTEIN** 16g

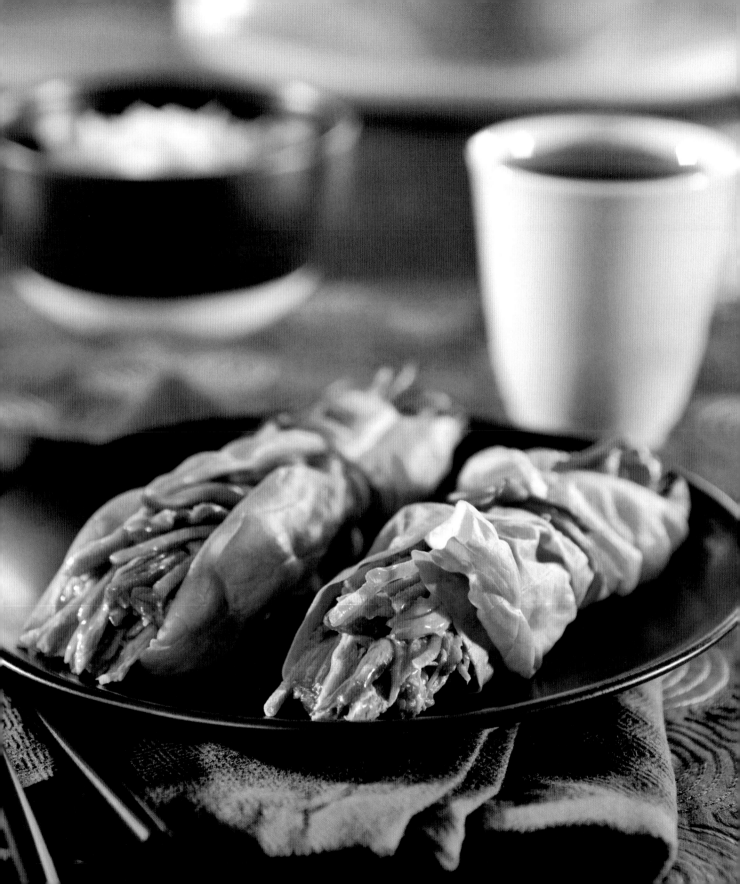

Chicken

3 tablespoons olive oil, divided

1 teaspoon salt

1 teaspoon dried oregano

1 teaspoon paprika

½ teaspoon black pepper

1 clove garlic, minced

1 pound chicken tenders, cut in half

Salad and Dressing

⅓ cup olive oil

3 tablespoons red wine vinegar

1 clove garlic, minced

Salt and black pepper

1 cup grape tomatoes, halved

1 cucumber, halved crosswise and cut into sticks

1 red bell pepper, sliced

2 avocados, thinly sliced

2 radishes, thinly sliced

Leaf lettuce and arugula

Black and white sesame seeds (optional)

Chicken Salad Bowl

MAKES 4 SERVINGS

1 For chicken, combine 1 tablespoon oil, 1 teaspoon salt, oregano, paprika, ½ teaspoon black pepper and 1 clove garlic in large bowl. Add chicken; toss until well blended.

2 Heat remaining 2 tablespoons oil in large skillet over medium-high heat. Add chicken; cook 8 to 10 minutes or until no longer pink, turning once.

3 For dressing, whisk ⅓ cup oil, vinegar and 1 clove garlic in small bowl. Season to taste with salt and black pepper.

4 Place tomatoes, cucumber, bell pepper, avocados, radishes, lettuce and arugula in serving bowls; drizzle with dressing. Slice chicken and place on salads. Sprinkle with sesame seeds, if desired.

Nutrients Per Serving (¼ of total recipe)

CALORIES 570 **TOTAL FAT** 44g **CARBS** 18g **NET CARBS** 9g
DIETARY FIBER 9g **PROTEIN** 30g

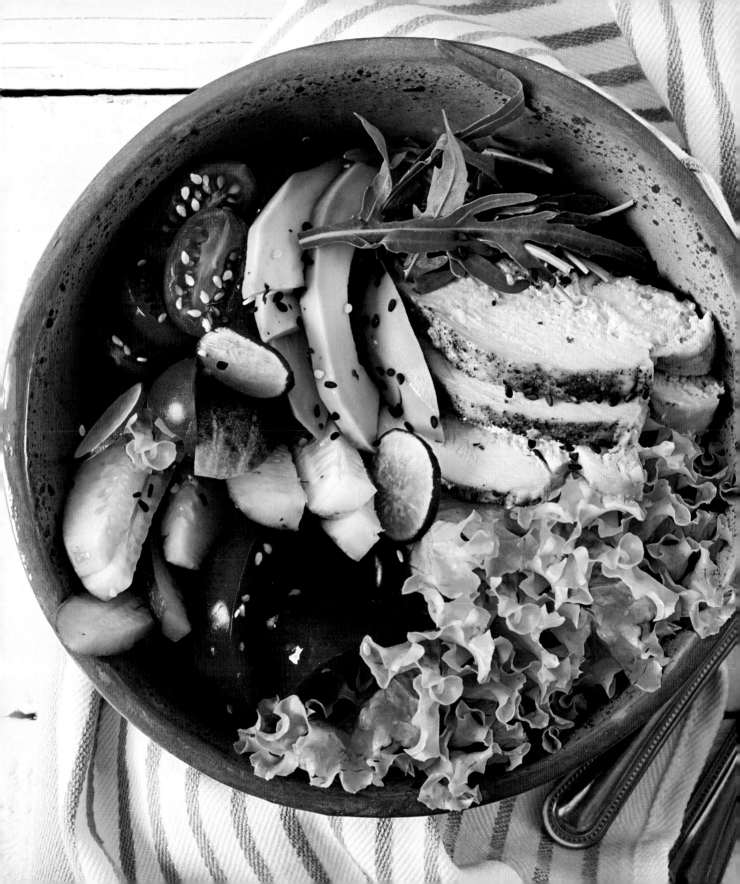

Garlic and Onion Sheet Pan Pizza
MAKES 16 SQUARES

2 teaspoons vegetable oil

1 head cauliflower (1½ pounds)

¾ cup almond flour

½ cup shredded Parmesan cheese

1½ cups (6 ounces) shredded mozzarella cheese, divided

1 teaspoon salt

1 clove garlic

½ teaspoon dried oregano

Black pepper

1 egg

¾ cup keto-friendly (sugar-free) marinara sauce

¼ cup whipping cream

½ sweet onion, halved and thinly sliced

1 tablespoon chopped garlic

1 Preheat oven to 425°F. Grease sheet pan with oil.

2 Break cauliflower into florets. Working in batches, pulse cauliflower in food processor until finely chopped. Measure 4 cups; place in large bowl. Reserve remaining cauliflower for another use. Add almond flour, Parmesan cheese, ½ cup mozzarella cheese, 1 teaspoon salt, 1 clove garlic and oregano. Season with black pepper; mix well. Add egg; mix with hands until thoroughly blended. Turn out onto prepared sheet pan; pat into 11×14-inch rectangle. Bake 20 minutes.

3 Remove crust from oven. Combine marinara sauce and cream in small bowl; spread over crust to within ½ inch of edges. Sprinkle evenly with onion, chopped garlic and remaining 1 cup mozzarella cheese. Bake 7 to 10 minutes or until cheese is bubbly and browned in spots. Cut into squares to serve.

Nutrients Per Serving (1 square)

CALORIES 120   **TOTAL FAT** 8g   **CARBS** 6g   **NET CARBS** 4g
DIETARY FIBER 2g   **PROTEIN** 6g

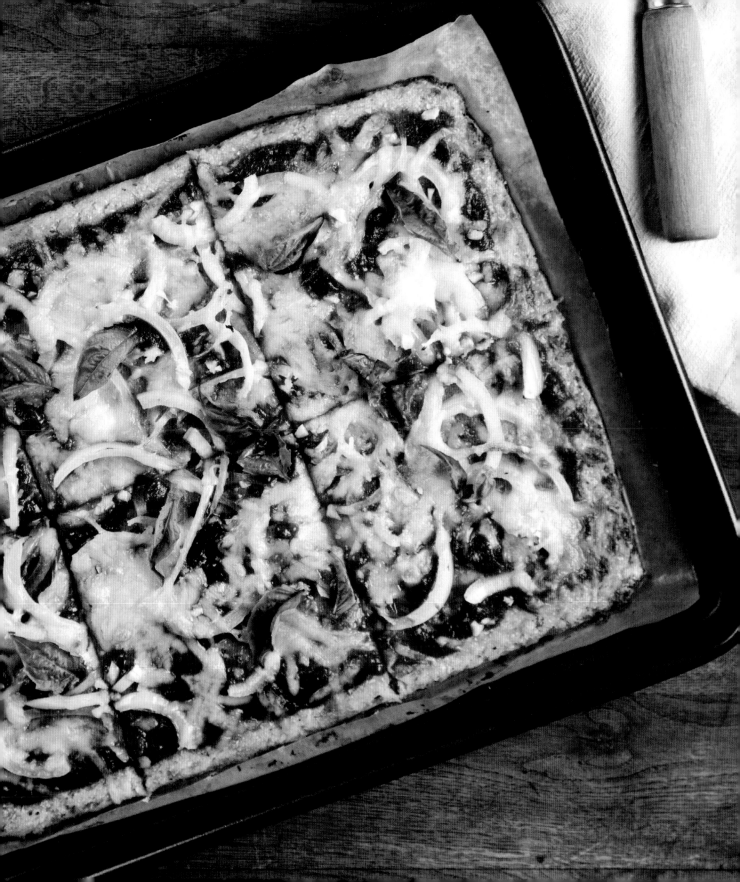

Zucchini Pizza Bites
MAKES 8 SERVINGS

1 medium zucchini

3 tablespoons pizza sauce

2 tablespoons tomato paste

¼ teaspoon dried oregano

¾ cup (3 ounces) shredded mozzarella cheese

¼ cup shredded Parmesan cheese

8 slices pitted black olives

8 slices pepperoni

1 Preheat broiler; set rack 4 inches from heat.

2 Trim and discard ends of zucchini. Cut zucchini into 16 (¼-inch-thick) diagonal slices. Place on nonstick baking sheet.

3 Combine pizza sauce, tomato paste and oregano in small bowl; mix well. Spread scant teaspoon sauce over each zucchini slice. Combine cheeses in small bowl. Top each zucchini slice with 1 tablespoon cheese mixture, pressing down into sauce. Place 1 olive slice on each of 8 pizza bites. Place 1 folded pepperoni slice on each remaining pizza bite.

4 Broil 3 minutes or until cheese is melted. Serve immediately.

Nutrients Per Serving (2 pizza bites)

CALORIES 75   **TOTAL FAT** 5g   **CARBS** 3g   **NET CARBS** 2g
DIETARY FIBER 1g   **PROTEIN** 5g

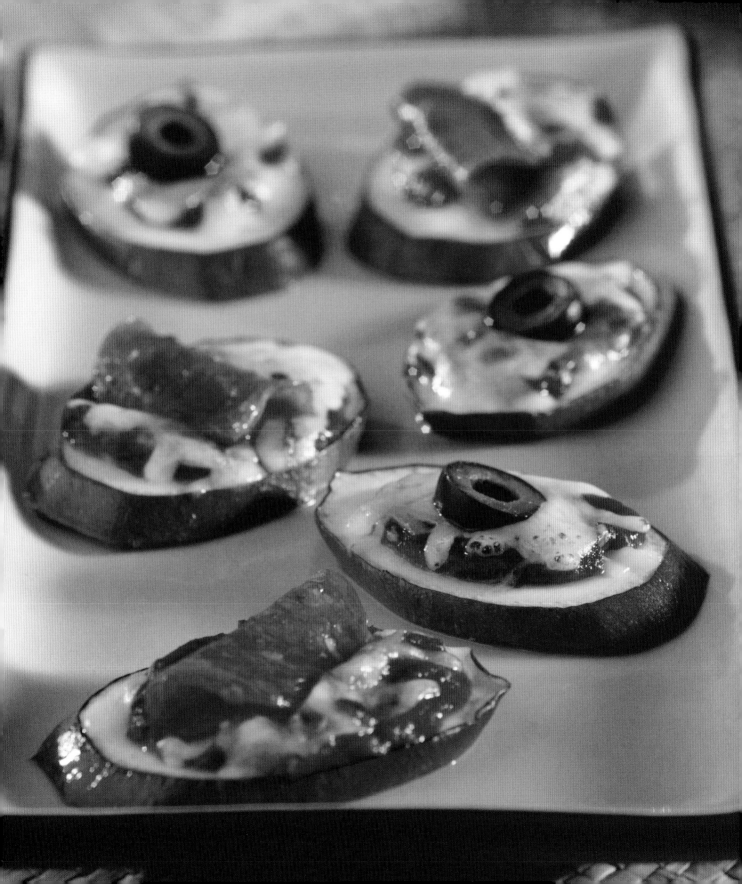

1 large poblano pepper

4 ounces smoked turkey breast, cut into 8 cubes

4 ounces pepper jack cheese, cut into 8 cubes

¼ cup salsa (optional)

Poblano Pepper Kabobs

MAKES 4 SERVINGS

1 Preheat oven to 400°F. Fill medium saucepan half full with water; bring to a boil over medium-high heat. Add poblano; cook 1 minute. Drain. Core, seed and cut poblano into 8 bite-size pieces.

2 Thread 1 piece of poblano, 1 piece of turkey and 1 piece of cheese onto each skewer. Repeat, ending with cheese.

3 Place kabobs on baking sheet. Bake 3 minutes or until cheese starts to melt. Serve with salsa, if desired.

Nutrients Per Serving (1 kabob)

CALORIES 145   **TOTAL FAT** 9g   **CARBS** 3g   **NET CARBS** 2g
DIETARY FIBER 1g   **PROTEIN** 13g

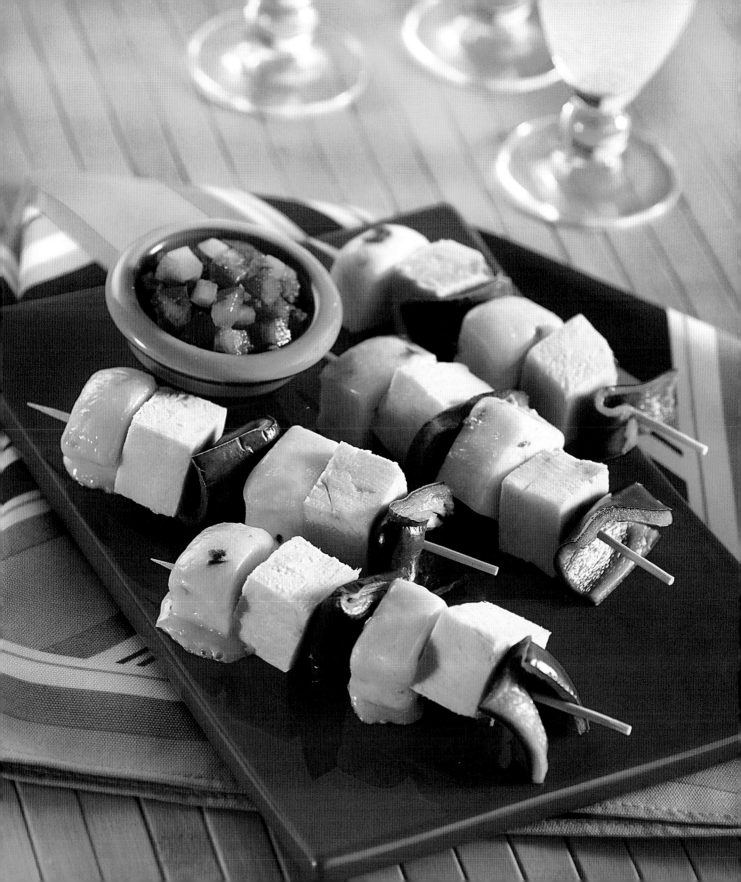

Southwestern Tuna Salad
MAKES 4 SERVINGS

2 limes, juiced, divided

12 ounces raw tuna steaks (about 1 inch thick)

1 pint cherry or grape tomatoes, halved

¼ cup diced ripe avocado (¼ of medium avocado)

1 jalapeño pepper, seeded and minced

1 green onion, chopped (green parts only)

1 tablespoon chopped fresh cilantro

1½ teaspoons canola oil

¼ teaspoon salt

¼ teaspoon ground cumin

⅛ teaspoon black pepper

Lime wedges (optional)

1 Place juice of 1 lime in glass baking dish or shallow bowl. Add tuna steaks. Marinate at room temperature 30 minutes, turning once.

2 Spray stovetop grill pan with nonstick cooking spray; heat over medium heat 30 seconds. Add tuna steaks; cook 5 to 6 minutes per side. Remove and set aside until cooled to room temperature. Cut into 1-inch pieces.

3 Combine tomatoes, avocado, jalapeño, green onion and cilantro in large bowl. Add tuna.

4 Whisk oil, remaining lime juice, salt, cumin and black pepper in small bowl. Pour over salad; toss to coat. Garnish with lime wedges.

Nutrients Per Serving (1 cup)
CALORIES 180 **TOTAL FAT** 7g **CARBS** 8g **NET CARBS** 5g
DIETARY FIBER 3g **PROTEIN** 21g

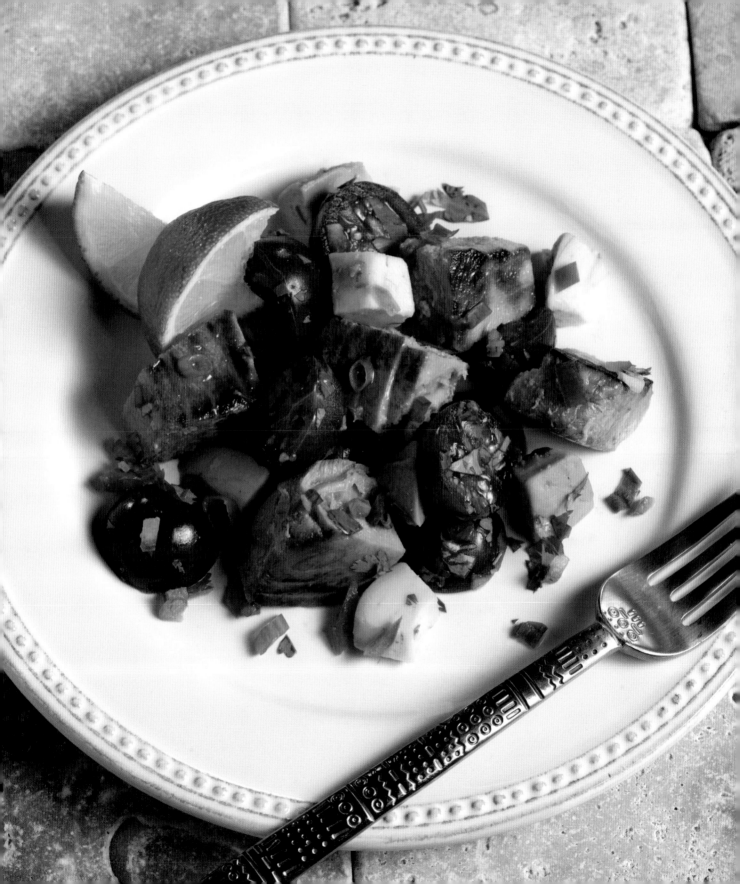

Ham and Cheese "Sushi" Rolls
MAKES 8 SERVINGS (64 PIECES)

4 thin slices deli ham (about 4×4 inches)

1 package (8 ounces) cream cheese, softened

1 piece (4 inches long) seedless cucumber, quartered lengthwise (about ½ cucumber)

4 thin slices (about 4×4 inches) American or Cheddar cheese, at room temperature

1 red bell pepper, cut into thin 4-inch-long strips

1 For ham sushi, pat 1 ham slice with paper towel to remove excess moisture and place on cutting board. Spread 2 tablespoons cream cheese to edges of ham slice. Pat 1 cucumber piece with paper towel to remove excess moisture; place at edge of ham slice. Roll up tightly, pressing gently to seal. Wrap in plastic wrap; refrigerate. Repeat with remaining ham slices, cream cheese and cucumber pieces.

2 For cheese sushi, spread 2 tablespoons cream cheese to edges of 1 cheese slice. Place 2 red pepper strips at edge of cheese slice. Roll up tightly, pressing gently to seal. Wrap in plastic wrap; refrigerate. Repeat with remaining cheese slices, cream cheese and red pepper strips.

3 To serve, remove plastic wrap from ham and cheese rolls. Cut each roll into ½-inch pieces.

Nutrients Per Serving (8 pieces)
CALORIES 145   **TOTAL FAT** 13g   **CARBS** 3g   **NET CARBS** 2g
DIETARY FIBER 1g   **PROTEIN** 5g

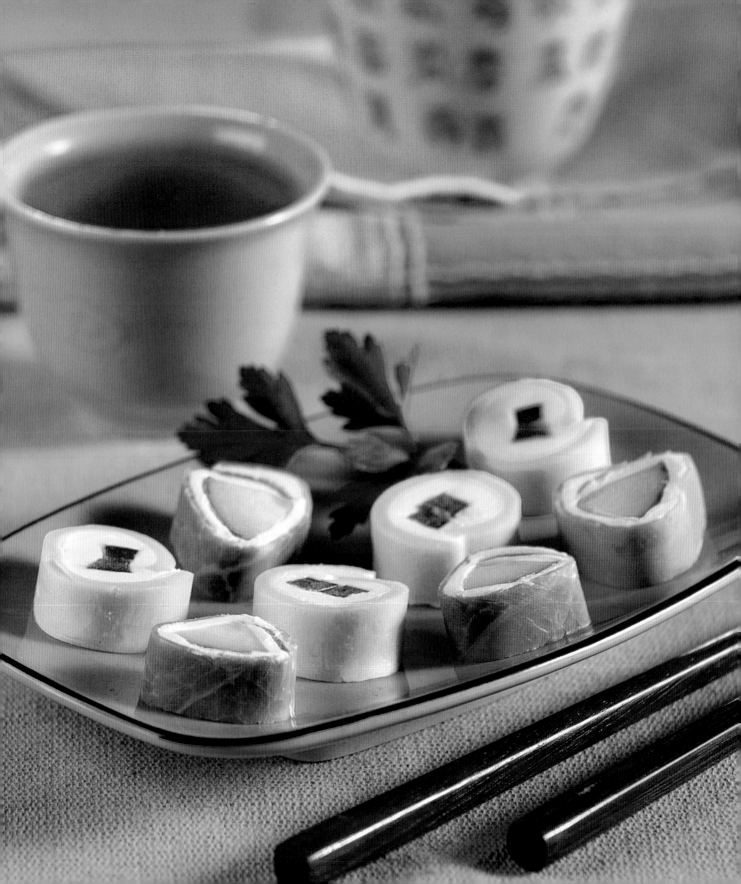

2 tablespoons
     horseradish
     mayonnaise
2 thin slices roast beef
     (1 ounce)
¼ cup crumbled blue
     cheese
¼ cup sliced red onion

Roast Beef Roll-Ups
MAKES 2 SERVINGS

1 Spread mayonnaise on roast beef slice. Sprinkle with blue cheese; layer with onion slices.

2 Roll up roast beef slice from short ends.

Nutrients Per Serving (1 roll-up)

CALORIES 80   **TOTAL FAT** 5g   **CARBS** 2g   **NET CARBS** 1g
DIETARY FIBER 1g   **PROTEIN** 6g

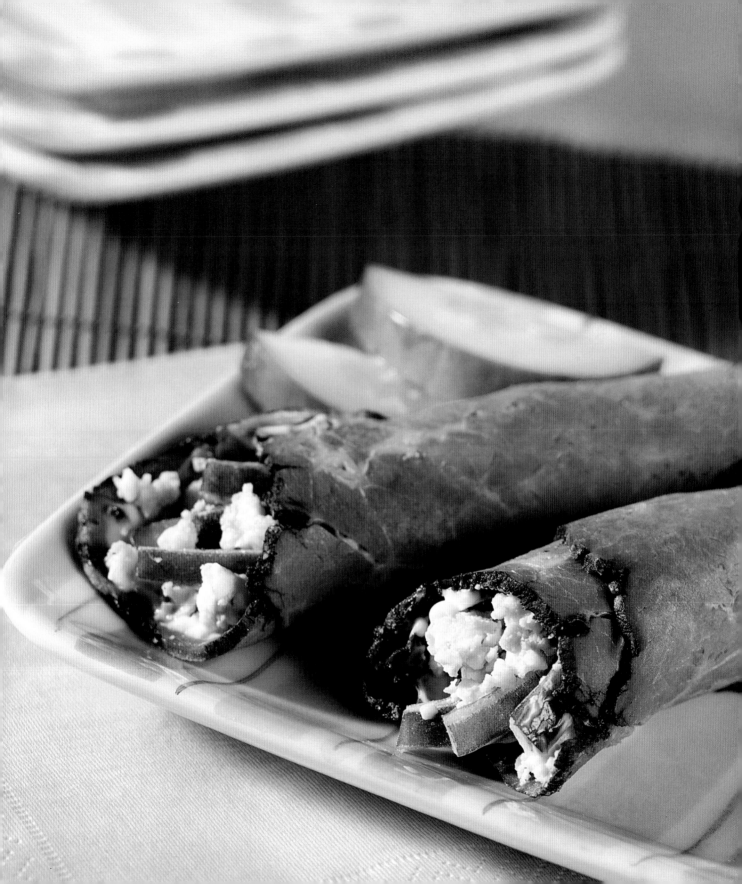

3 large ripe avocados, halved and pitted

6 tablespoons lemon juice

¾ cup mayonnaise

1½ tablespoons grated onion

¼ teaspoon celery salt

¼ teaspoon garlic powder

Salt and black pepper

2 cups diced cooked chicken

½ cup (2 ounces) shredded sharp Cheddar cheese

Minced fresh chives (optional)

Chicken Avocado Boats
MAKES 6 SERVINGS

1 Preheat oven to 350°F. Sprinkle each avocado half with 1 tablespoon lemon juice.

2 Combine mayonnaise, onion, celery salt, garlic powder, salt and pepper in medium bowl. Stir in chicken; mix well.

3 Drain any excess lemon juice from avocado halves. Fill avocado halves with chicken mixture; sprinkle with cheese.

4 Arrange filled avocado halves in single layer in baking dish. Pour water into baking dish to depth of ½ inch. Bake 15 minutes or until cheese melts. Garnish with chives.

Nutrients Per Serving (1 filled avocado half)

CALORIES 490   **TOTAL FAT** 42g   **CARBS** 11g   **NET CARBS** 4g
DIETARY FIBER 7g   **PROTEIN** 20g

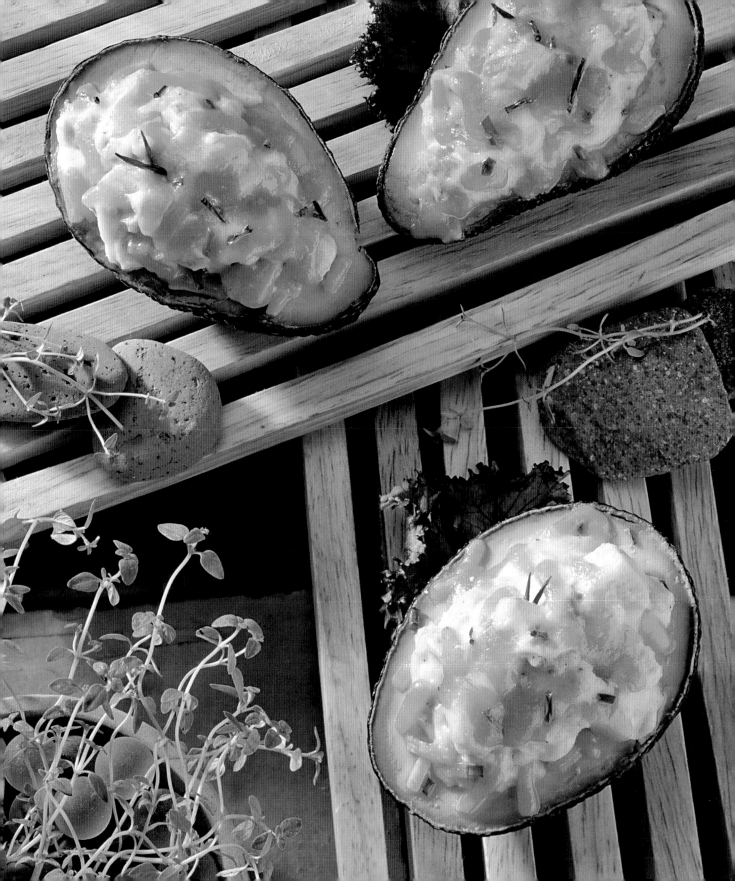

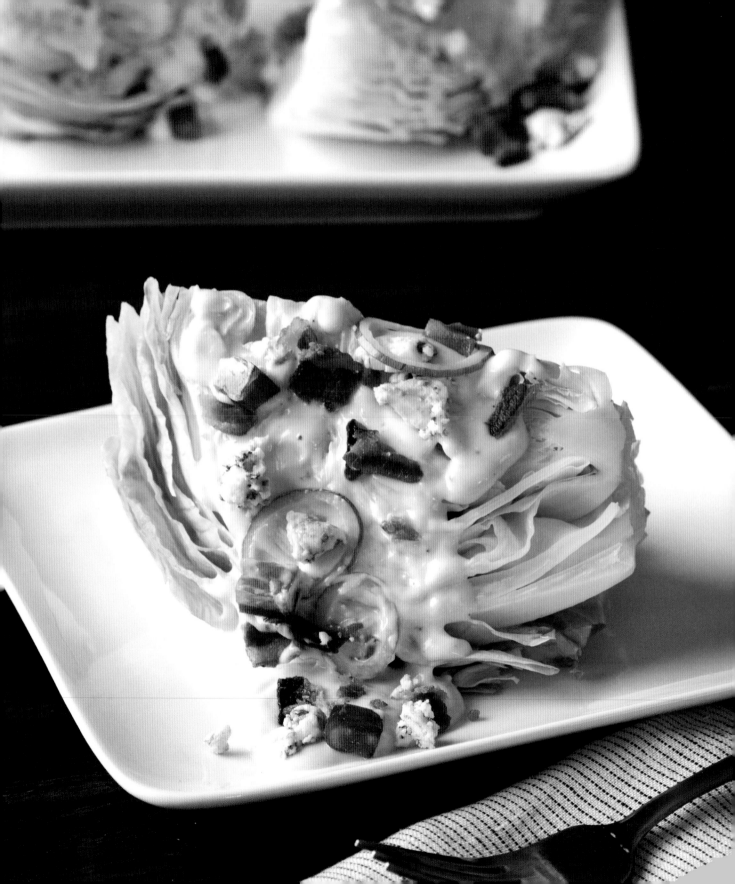

Salads

Wedge Salad

MAKES 4 SERVINGS

1 For dressing, combine mayonnaise, buttermilk, ½ cup cheese, garlic, onion powder, salt and pepper in food processor or blender; process until smooth.

2 For salad, cut lettuce into quarters through stem end; remove stem from each wedge. Place wedges on individual serving plates; top with dressing. Sprinkle with tomato, onion, remaining ½ cup cheese and bacon.

Nutrients Per Serving (¼ of total recipe)

CALORIES 460   **TOTAL FAT** 42g   **CARBS** 9g   **NET CARBS** 7g
DIETARY FIBER 2g   **PROTEIN** 13g

Dressing

- ¾ cup mayonnaise
- ½ cup buttermilk
- 1 cup crumbled blue cheese, divided
- 1 clove garlic, minced
- ⅛ teaspoon onion powder
- ⅛ teaspoon salt
- ⅛ teaspoon ground black pepper

Salad

- 1 head iceberg lettuce
- 1 large tomato, diced (about 1 cup)
- ½ small red onion, cut into thin rings
- ½ cup crumbled crisp-cooked bacon (6 slices)

Pickled Onions

- 1 cup thinly sliced red onion
- ½ cup white wine vinegar
- ¼ cup water
- 1 teaspoon salt

Dressing

- 1 cup mayonnaise
- 1 cup fresh Italian parsley leaves
- 1 cup baby arugula
- ¼ cup extra virgin olive oil
- 3 tablespoons lemon juice
- 3 tablespoons minced fresh chives
- 2 tablespoons fresh tarragon leaves
- 1 clove garlic, minced
- 1 teaspoon Dijon mustard
- ½ teaspoon salt
- ⅛ teaspoon black pepper

Salad

- 4 eggs
- 4 cups Italian salad blend (romaine and radicchio)
- 2 cups chopped stemmed kale
- 2 cups baby arugula
- 2 avocados, halved and sliced
- 2 tomatoes, cut into wedges
- 2 cups cooked chicken strips
- 1 cup chopped crisp-cooked bacon

Green Goddess Cobb Salad

MAKES 6 SERVINGS

1 For pickled onions, combine onion, vinegar, ¼ cup water and 1 teaspoon salt in large glass jar. Seal jar; shake well. Refrigerate at least 1 hour or up to 1 week.

2 For dressing, combine mayonnaise, parsley, 1 cup arugula, oil, lemon juice, chives, tarragon, garlic, mustard, ½ teaspoon salt and pepper in food processor; blend until smooth, stopping to scrape down side once or twice. Transfer to jar; refrigerate until ready to use. Just before serving, stir in 1 to 2 tablespoons water, if necessary, to reach desired consistency.

3 Fill medium saucepan with water; bring to a boil over high heat. Carefully lower eggs into water. Reduce heat to medium; boil gently 12 minutes. Drain eggs; add cold water and ice cubes to saucepan to cool eggs. When eggs are cool, peel and cut in half lengthwise or cut into wedges.

4 For salad, combine salad blend, kale, 2 cups arugula and pickled onions in large bowl; divide among six serving bowls. Top with avocados, tomatoes, chicken, bacon and eggs. Top with ¼ cup dressing; toss to coat.

Nutrients Per Serving (⅙ of total recipe)

CALORIES 750 **TOTAL FAT** 62g **CARBS** 14g **NET CARBS** 8g
DIETARY FIBER 6g **PROTEIN** 40g

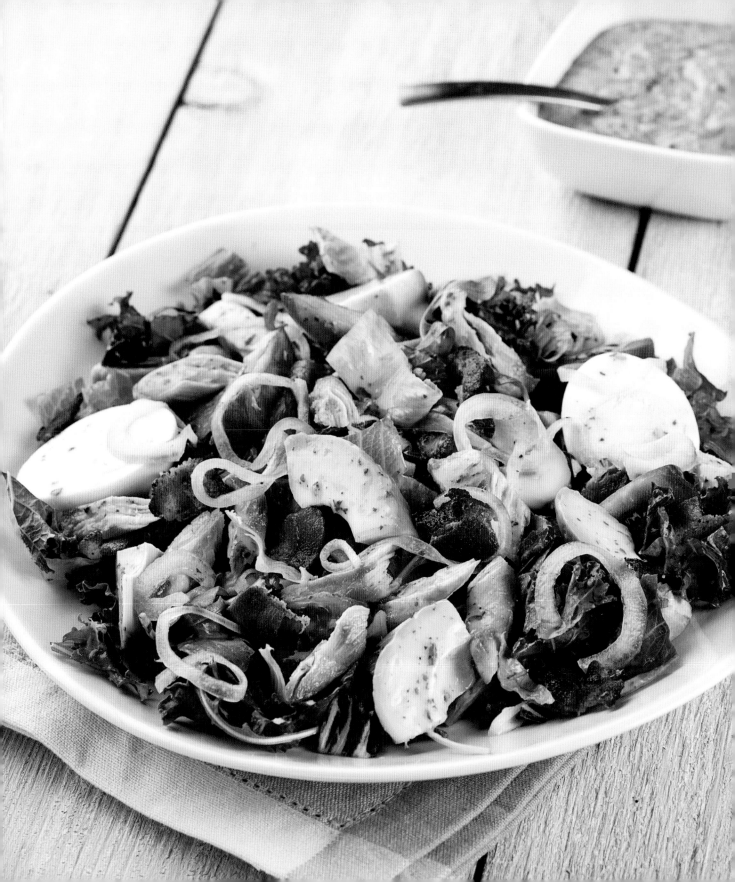

Salad

3 medium tomatoes, cut into 8 wedges each

1 green bell pepper, cut into 1-inch pieces

½ English cucumber, quartered lengthwise and sliced crosswise

½ red onion, thinly sliced

½ cup pitted kalamata olives

1 block (8 ounces) feta cheese, cut into ½-inch cubes

Dressing

6 tablespoons extra virgin olive oil

3 tablespoons red wine vinegar

1 to 2 cloves garlic, minced

¾ teaspoon dried oregano

¾ teaspoon salt

¼ teaspoon black pepper

Greek Salad
MAKES 6 SERVINGS

1 Combine tomatoes, bell pepper, cucumber, onion and olives in large bowl. Top with cheese.

2 For dressing, whisk oil, vinegar, garlic, oregano, salt and black pepper in medium bowl until well blended. Pour over salad; stir gently to coat.

Nutrients Per Serving (⅙ of total recipe)

CALORIES 233 TOTAL FAT 21g CARBS 7g NET CARBS 6g
DIETARY FIBER 1g PROTEIN 8g

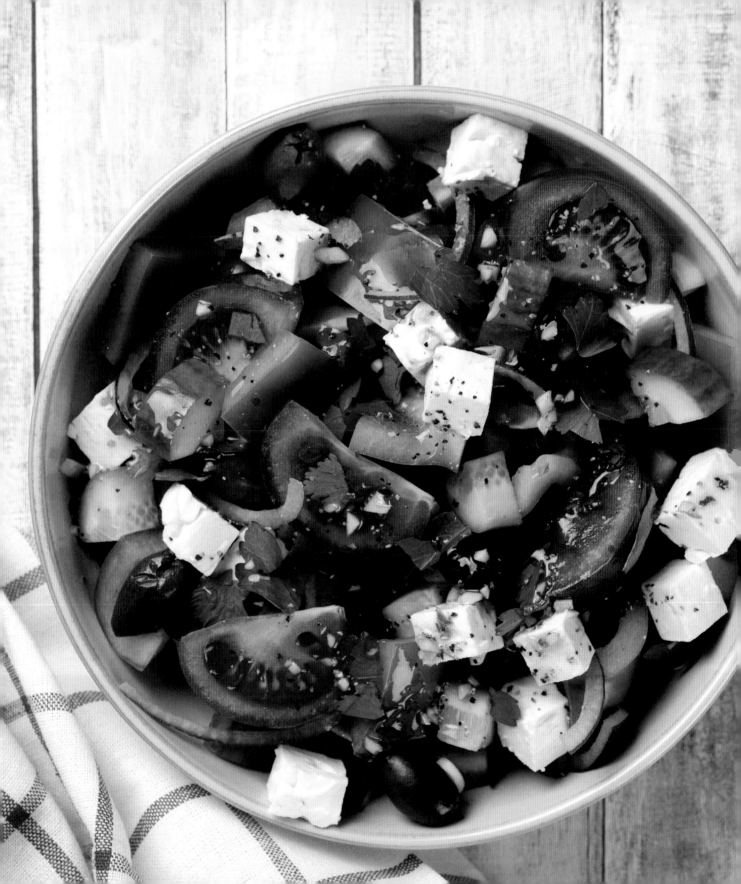

Dressing

⅓ cup red wine vinegar

2 cloves garlic, minced

1 teaspoon Italian seasoning

¼ teaspoon salt

¼ teaspoon black pepper

⅓ cup olive oil

Salad

1 package (5 ounces) spring mix

5 romaine lettuce leaves, chopped

1 small cucumber, diced

2 small plum tomatoes, diced

½ red onion, thinly sliced

¼ cup pitted kalamata olives

4 radishes, thinly sliced

4 ounces thinly sliced Genoa salami, cut into ¼-inch strips

4 ounces provolone cheese, cut into ¼-inch strips

¼ cup grated Parmesan cheese

Garbage Salad

MAKES 4 SERVINGS

1 For dressing, whisk vinegar, garlic, Italian seasoning, salt and pepper in small bowl until blended. Slowly whisk in oil in thin steady stream until well blended.

2 Combine spring mix, romaine, cucumber, tomatoes, onion, olives and radishes in large bowl. Add half of dressing; toss gently to coat. Top with salami and provolone cheese; sprinkle with Parmesan cheese. Serve with remaining dressing.

Nutrients Per Serving (¼ of total recipe)

CALORIES 420 **TOTAL FAT** 35g **CARBS** 10g **NET CARBS** 7g
DIETARY FIBER 3g **PROTEIN** 19g

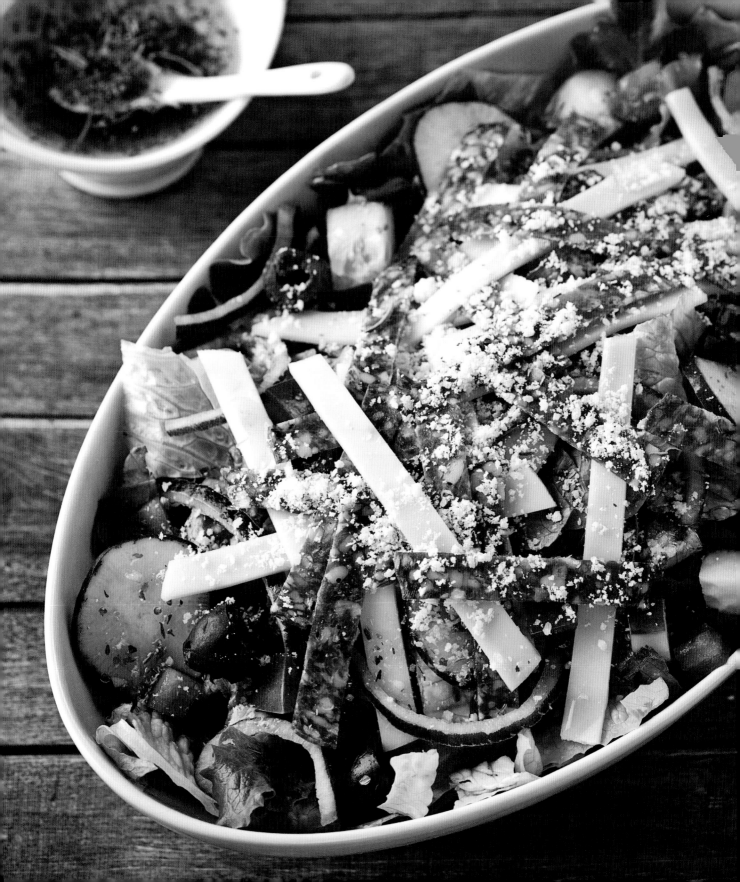

2 teaspoons salt

1 head cauliflower, cut into 1-inch florets

¾ cup mayonnaise

1 tablespoon yellow mustard

2 tablespoons minced fresh parsley

⅓ cup chopped dill pickle

⅓ cup minced red onion

2 hard-cooked eggs, chopped

Salt and black pepper

Cauliflower Picnic Salad
MAKES 6 SERVINGS

1 Fill large saucepan with 1 inch of water. Bring to a simmer over medium-high heat; stir in salt. Add cauliflower; reduce heat to medium. Cover and cook 5 to 7 minutes or until cauliflower is fork-tender but not mushy. Drain and cool slightly.

2 Whisk mayonnaise, mustard and parsley in large bowl. Stir in pickle and onion. Gently fold in cauliflower and eggs. Season with salt and pepper.

Nutrients Per Serving (⅙ of total recipe)

CALORIES 240   TOTAL FAT 22g   CARBS 8g   NET CARBS 5g
DIETARY FIBER 3g   PROTEIN 5g

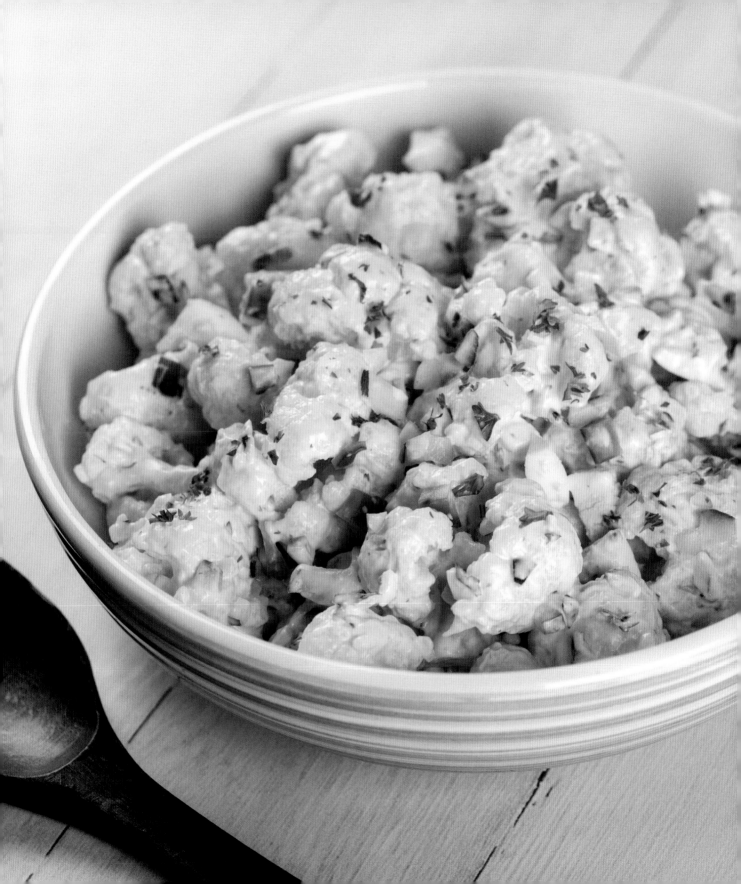

1 package (10 ounces)
    torn mixed salad
    greens *or* 8 cups
    torn romaine lettuce

6 ounces deli chicken,
    turkey or smoked
    turkey breast, diced

1 large tomato, seeded
    and chopped

⅓ cup crisp-cooked and
    crumbled bacon

1 large ripe avocado,
    diced

Crumbled blue cheese

Keto-friendly blue
    cheese or Caesar
    salad dressing

Classic Cobb Salad

MAKES 4 SERVINGS

1 Place salad greens in serving bowl. Top with chicken,
   tomato, bacon and avocado in rows.

2 Sprinkle with blue cheese. Serve with dressing.

Nutrients Per Serving (1 cup salad)

CALORIES 222   **TOTAL FAT** 13g   **CARBS** 12g   **NET CARBS** 9g
DIETARY FIBER 3g   **PROTEIN** 17g

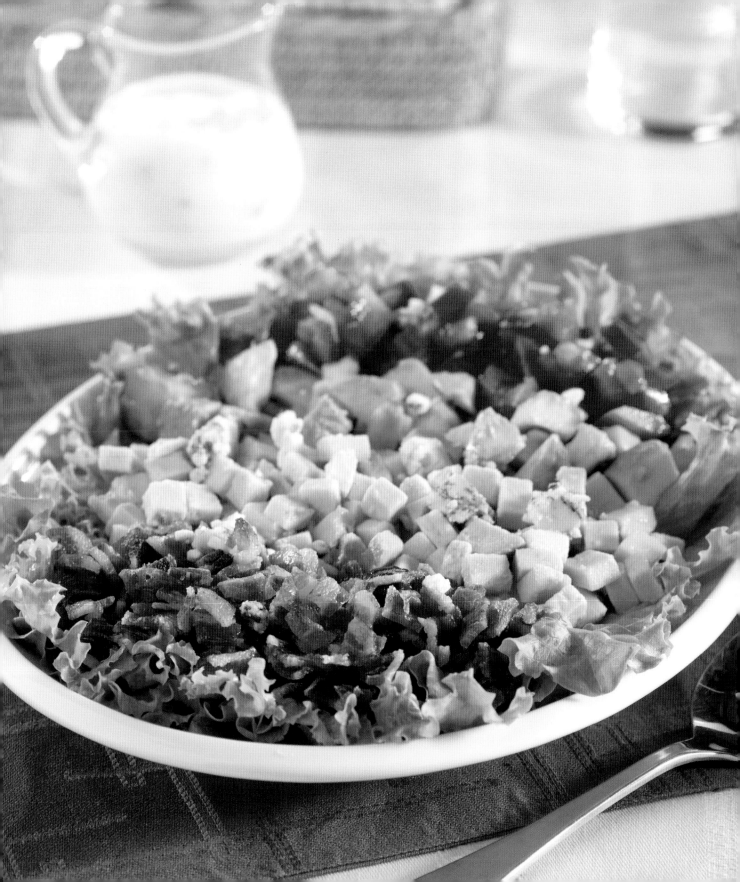

1 pound ground beef

½ cup chopped onion

2 cloves garlic, minced

1 teaspoon ground cumin

1 teaspoon chili powder

½ teaspoon salt

½ cup salsa, divided

6 cups packed torn or sliced romaine lettuce

1 large tomato, chopped

1 cup (4 ounces) shredded Mexican cheese blend or taco cheese, divided

2 tablespoons canola oil

1 ripe avocado, diced

¼ cup sour cream

Taco Salad Supreme

MAKES 4 SERVINGS

1 Brown beef and onion in large skillet over medium-high heat 6 to 8 minutes, stirring to break up meat. Drain fat. Add garlic, cumin, chili powder and salt; cook 1 minute, stirring frequently. Stir in ¼ cup salsa; cook and stir 1 minute. Remove from heat.

2 Combine lettuce, tomato, ½ cup cheese, remaining ¼ cup salsa and oil in large bowl. Divide salad among two serving plates. Spoon meat mixture evenly over salads; top with remaining ½ cup cheese, avocado and sour cream.

Nutrients Per Serving

(2 cups salad with ⅔ cup meat mixture, 2 tablespoons cheese and 1 tablespoon sour cream)

CALORIES 584   **TOTAL FAT** 47g   **CARBS** 11g   **NET CARBS** 6g
DIETARY FIBER 5g   **PROTEIN** 30g

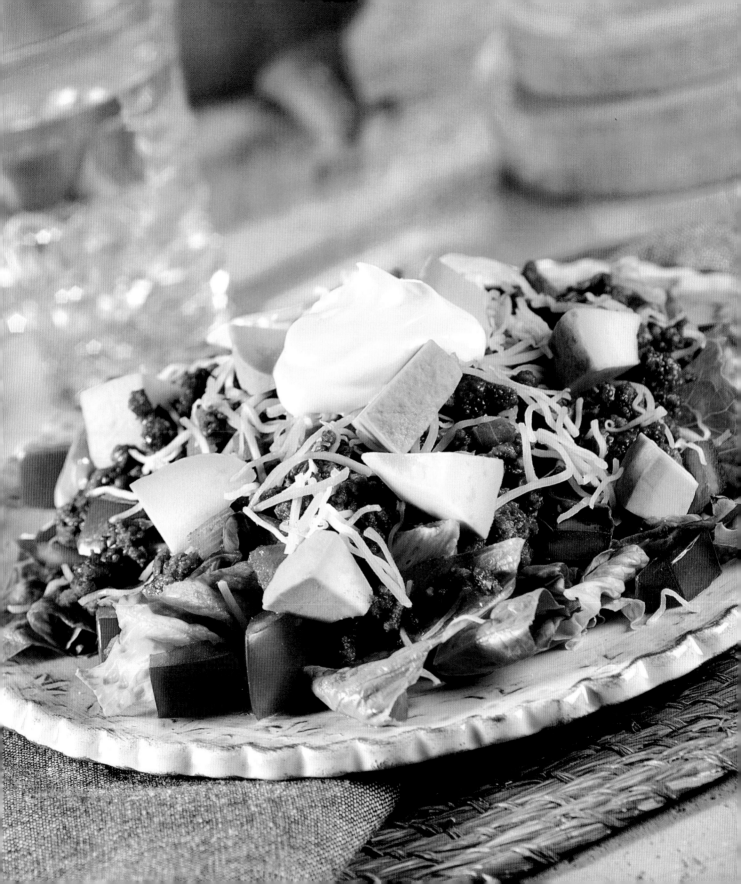

½ cup red wine vinegar

¼ cup olive oil

1 teaspoon salt

1 teaspoon Dijon mustard

½ teaspoon dried oregano

1 clove garlic, minced

¼ teaspoon black pepper

2 cups small cauliflower florets (½ inch)

1 head iceberg lettuce, chopped

1 container crumbled blue cheese

1 pint grape tomatoes, halved *or* 1 cup finely chopped tomatoes

½ cup finely chopped red onion

2 green onions, finely chopped

1 avocado, diced

Cauliflower Chopped Salad

MAKES 8 SERVINGS

1 For cauliflower, whisk vinegar, oil, salt, mustard, oregano, garlic and pepper in medium bowl. Add cauliflower; stir to coat. Cover and refrigerate several hours or overnight.

2 For salad, combine lettuce, blue cheese, tomatoes, red onion and green onions in large bowl; toss to coat. Remove cauliflower from marinade using slotted spoon; place on salad. Whisk marinade; pour over salad and toss to coat. Top with avocado; mix gently.

Nutrients Per Serving (⅛ of total recipe)

CALORIES 190 **TOTAL FAT** 15g **CARBS** 12g **NET CARBS** 8g
DIETARY FIBER 4g **PROTEIN** 5g

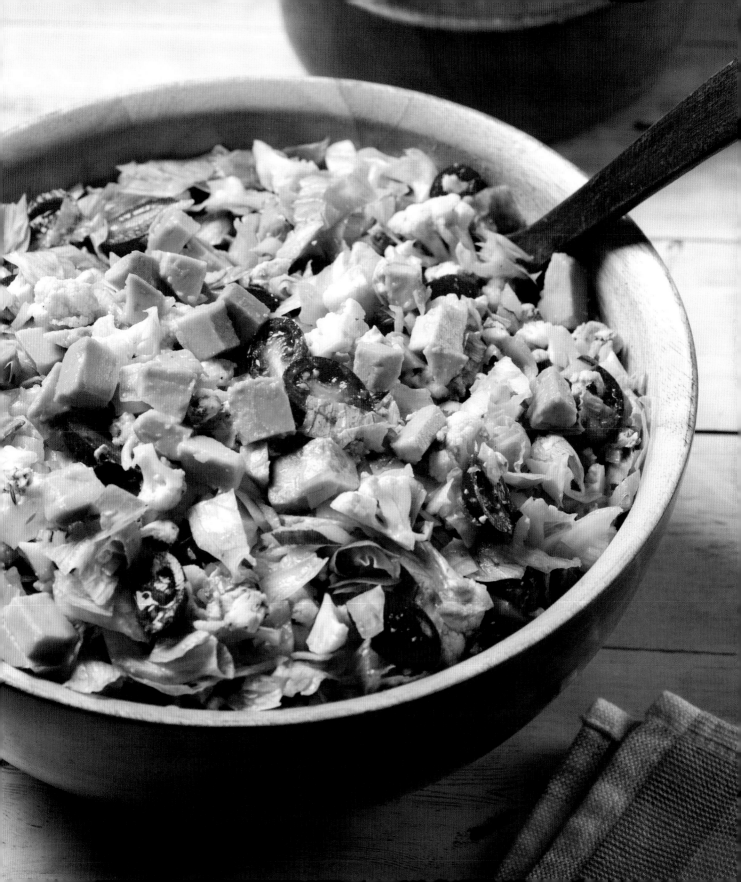

Basil Vinaigrette

- 3 tablespoons olive oil
- 1 tablespoon white wine vinegar
- 1 tablespoon minced fresh basil
- 1 clove garlic, minced
- 1 teaspoon minced fresh chives
- ¼ teaspoon salt
- ¼ teaspoon black pepper

Salad

- 1¼ teaspoons salt, divided
- 1 pound asparagus, trimmed
- 1 pound salmon fillet
- 1½ teaspoons olive oil
- ¼ teaspoon black pepper
- 4 lemon wedges

Salmon Salad with Basil Vinaigrette
MAKES 4 SERVINGS

1 For vinaigrette, whisk 3 tablespoons oil, vinegar, basil, garlic, chives, ¼ teaspoon salt and ¼ teaspoon pepper in small bowl until well blended.

2 Preheat oven to 400°F or prepare grill for direct cooking.

3 Combine 3 inches of water and 1 teaspoon salt in large saucepan; bring to boil over high heat. Add asparagus; simmer 6 to 8 minutes or until crisp-tender; drain and set aside.

4 Brush salmon with 1½ teaspoons oil. Sprinkle with remaining ¼ teaspoon salt and ¼ teaspoon pepper. Place fish in shallow baking pan; cook 11 to 13 minutes or until center is opaque. (Or grill on well-oiled grid over medium-high heat 4 or 5 minutes per side or until center is opaque.)

5 Remove skin from salmon; break into bite-size pieces. Arrange salmon over asparagus; drizzle with vinaigrette. Serve with lemon wedges.

Nutrients Per Serving (1½ cups)

CALORIES 332 **TOTAL FAT** 24g **CARBS** 5g **NET CARBS** 3g
DIETARY FIBER 2g **PROTEIN** 25g

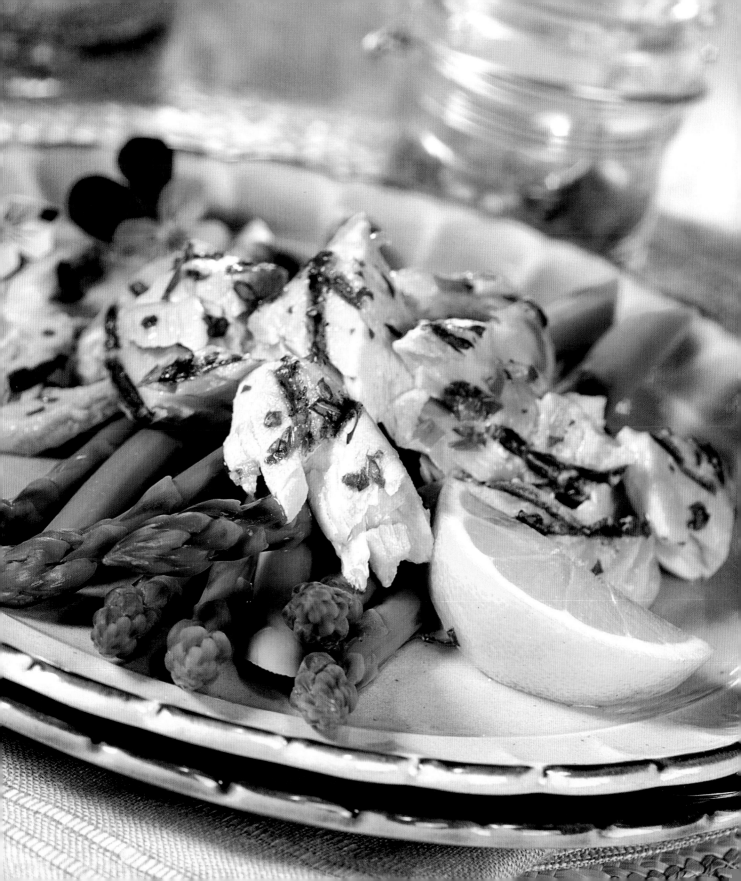

1 head cauliflower, cut into florets and thinly sliced

¾ cup balsamic vinegar

½ cup olive oil

1 teaspoon salt

1 clove garlic, minced

1 teaspoon Italian seasoning

1 container (8 ounces) pearl-shaped fresh mozzarella cheese *or* 1 (8-ounce) ball fresh mozzarella, sliced or chopped

2 cups chopped fresh tomatoes *or* 1 pint grape tomatoes, halved

¼ cup shredded fresh basil

Cauliflower Caprese Salad
MAKES 8 SERVINGS

1 Place cauliflower in large resealable food storage bag or large bowl. Add vinegar, oil, salt, garlic and Italian seasoning. Seal bag; shake to coat. Marinate in refrigerator 8 hours or overnight.

2 Pour cauliflower and marinade into large bowl. Stir in cheese, tomatoes and basil.

Nutrients Per Serving (⅛ of total recipe)

CALORIES 250 **TOTAL FAT** 20g **CARBS** 10g **NET CARBS** 8g **DIETARY FIBER** 2g **PROTEIN** 7g

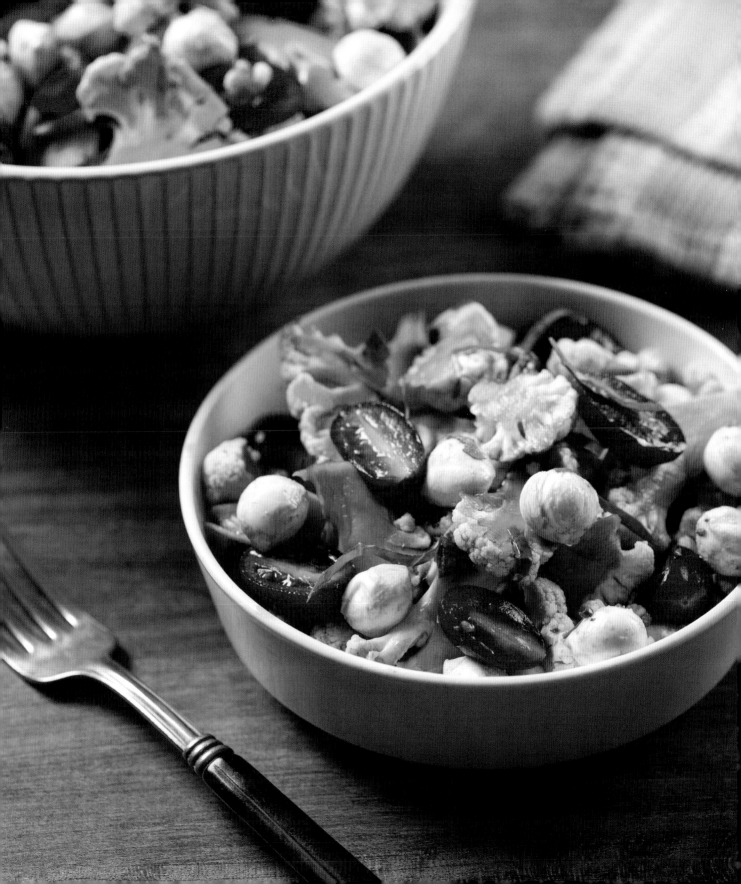

3 eggs

4 cups mixed baby salad greens

2 cups green beans, cut into 1½-inch pieces, cooked and drained

4 slices thick-cut bacon, crisp-cooked and crumbled

1 tablespoon minced fresh basil, chives or Italian parsley

3 tablespoons olive oil

1 tablespoon red wine vinegar

1 teaspoon Dijon mustard

¼ teaspoon salt

¼ teaspoon black pepper

Market Salad
MAKES 4 SERVINGS

1 Bring medium saucepan of water to a boil over high heat. Gently lower eggs into water; reduce heat to medium. Simmer 12 minutes. Drain eggs; add cold water and ice cubes to saucepan to cool eggs. Peel eggs and cut into wedges when cool enough to handle.

2 Combine salad greens, green beans, bacon and basil in large serving bowl. Add eggs. Whisk oil, vinegar, mustard, salt and pepper in small bowl until well blended. Drizzle dressing over salad; toss gently to coat.

Nutrients Per Serving (about 2 cups)
CALORIES 224   **TOTAL FAT** 18g   **CARBS** 7g   **NET CARBS** 4g
DIETARY FIBER 3g   **PROTEIN** 9g

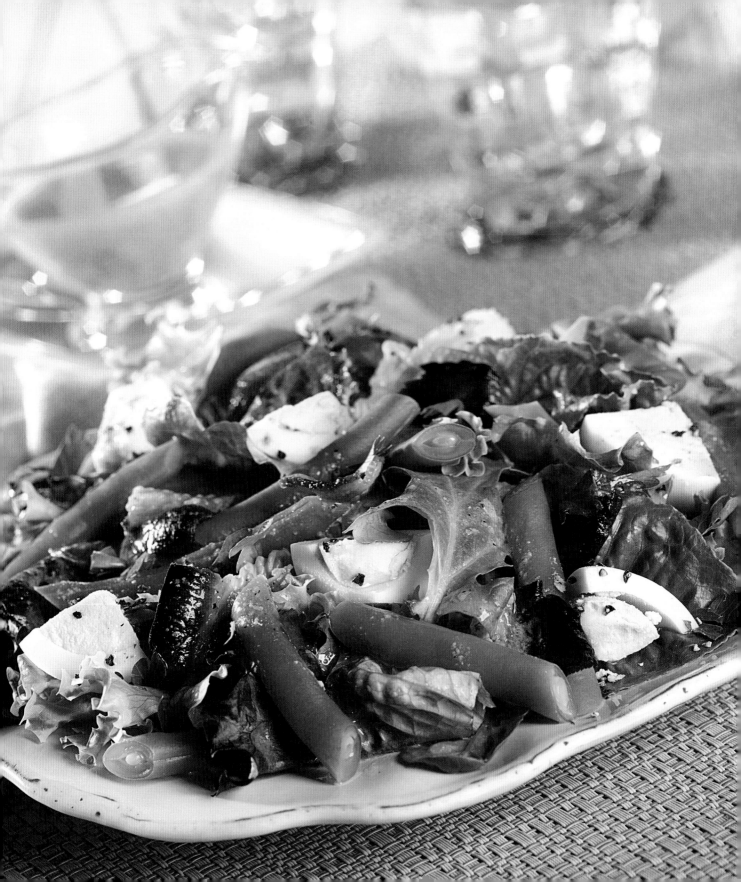

Tomato, Avocado and Cucumber Salad with Feta Cheese

MAKES 4 SERVINGS

1½ tablespoons extra virgin olive oil

1 tablespoon balsamic vinegar

1 clove garlic, minced

¼ teaspoon salt

¼ teaspoon black pepper

2 cups diced seeded plum tomatoes

1 small ripe avocado, diced into ½-inch chunks

½ cup chopped cucumber

⅓ cup crumbled feta cheese

4 large red leaf lettuce leaves

Chopped fresh basil (optional)

1 Whisk oil, vinegar, garlic, salt and pepper in medium bowl. Add tomatoes and avocado; toss gently to coat. Stir in cucumber and cheese.

2 Arrange 1 lettuce leaf on each serving plate. Spoon salad evenly onto lettuce leaves. Top with basil, if desired.

Nutrients Per Serving (¼ of total recipe)

CALORIES 138   **TOTAL FAT** 11g   **CARBS** 7g   **NET CARBS** 5g
DIETARY FIBER 2g   **PROTEIN** 4g

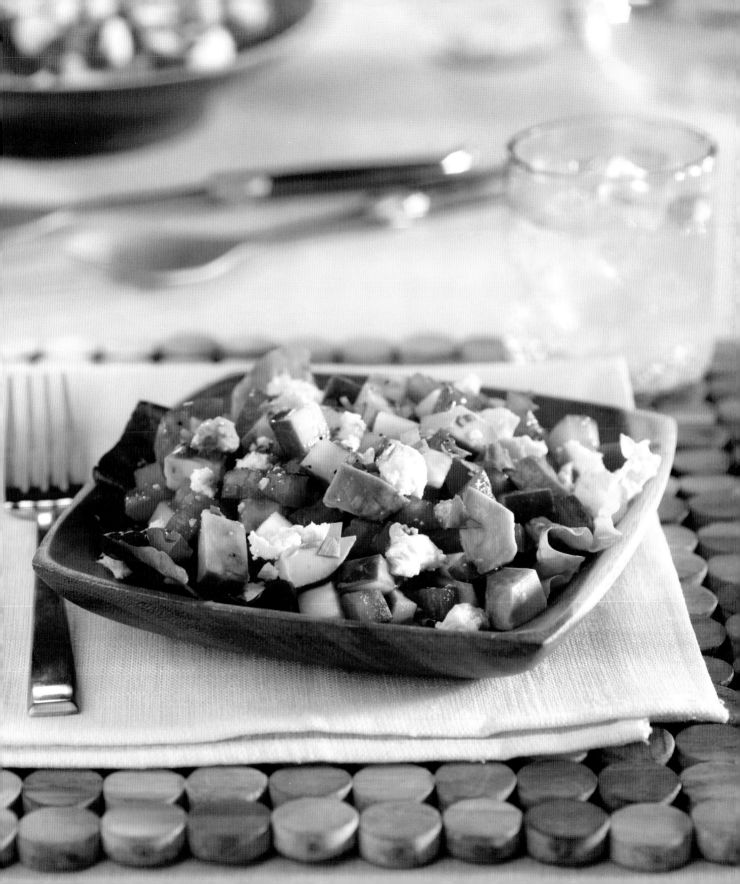

12 ounces coarsely flaked cooked crabmeat *or* 2 packages (6 ounces each) frozen crabmeat, thawed and drained

1 cup chopped tomatoes

1 cup sliced cucumber

⅓ cup sliced red onion

¼ cup mayonnaise

¼ cup sour cream

¼ cup chopped fresh parsley

2 tablespoons milk

2 teaspoons chopped fresh tarragon *or* ½ teaspoon dried tarragon

1 clove garlic, minced

¼ teaspoon hot pepper sauce

8 cups fresh baby spinach

Crab Spinach Salad with Tarragon Dressing
MAKES 4 SERVINGS

1 Combine crabmeat, tomatoes, cucumber and onion in medium bowl. Combine mayonnaise, sour cream, parsley, milk, tarragon, garlic and hot pepper sauce in small bowl.

2 Divide spinach among four salad plates or bowls. Place crabmeat mixture on spinach; drizzle with dressing.

Nutrients Per Serving
(1 cup salad with 1½ tablespoons dressing and 2 cups spinach)

CALORIES 170 **TOTAL FAT** 4g **CARBS** 14g **NET CARBS** 4g
DIETARY FIBER 10g **PROTEIN** 22g

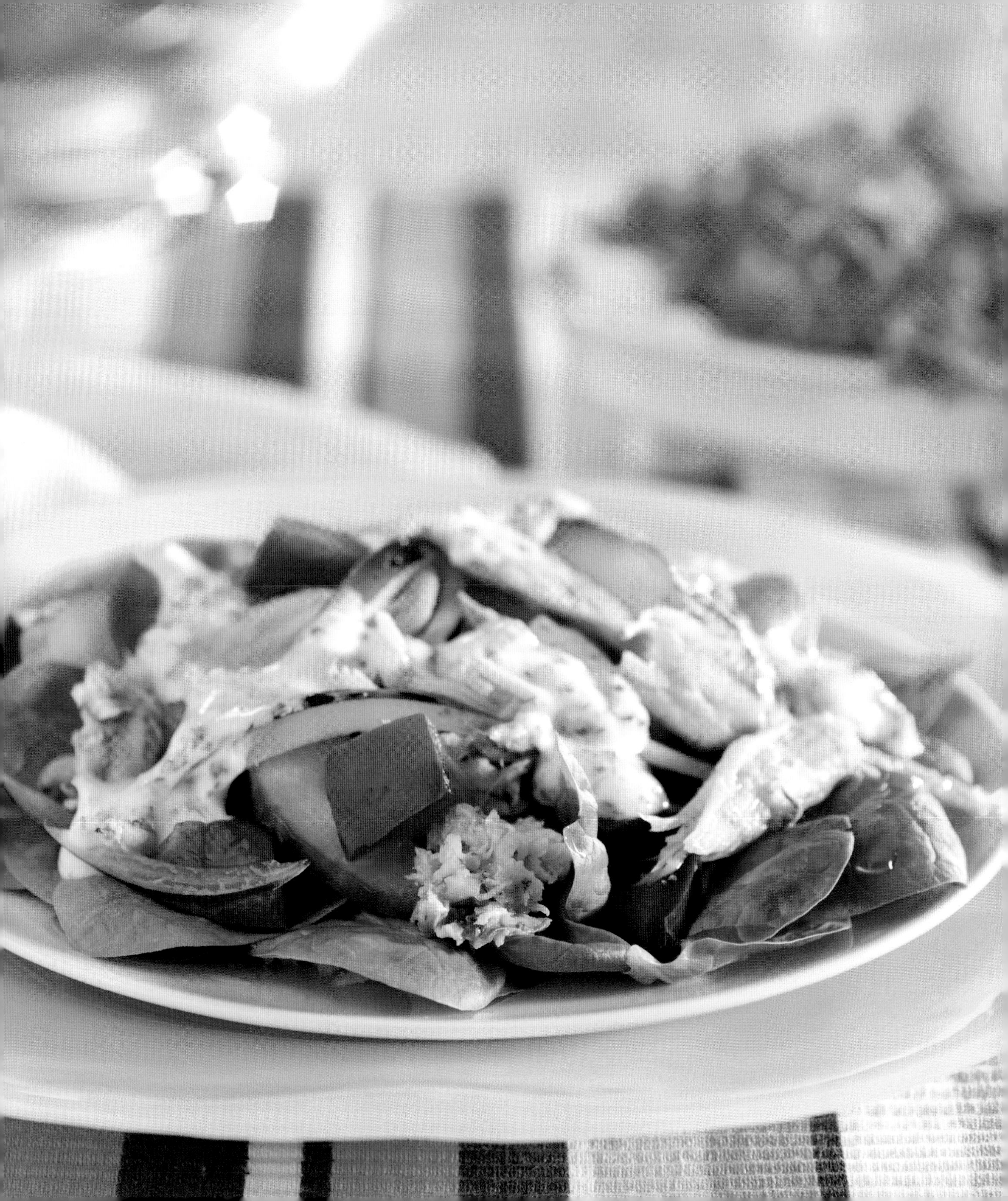

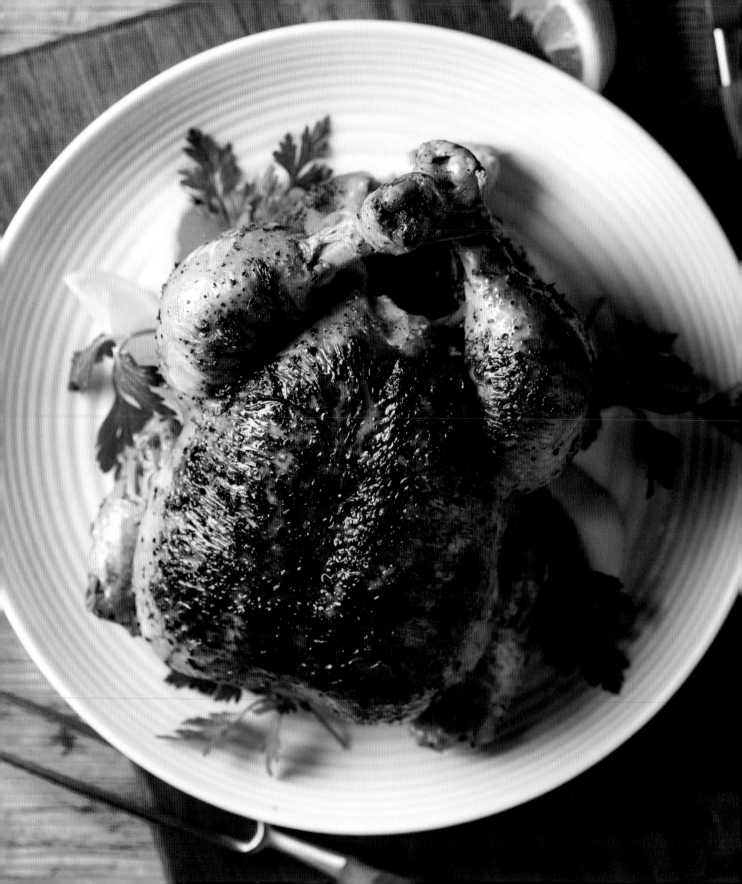

Poultry

Simple Roasted Chicken

MAKES 4 SERVINGS

1 Preheat oven to 425°F. Pat chicken dry; place in baking dish or baking pan.

2 Combine butter, salt, onion powder, thyme, garlic powder, paprika and pepper in small microwavable bowl; mash with fork until well blended. Loosen skin on breasts and thighs; spread about one third of butter mixture under skin.

3 Microwave remaining butter mixture until melted. Brush melted butter mixture all over outside of chicken and inside cavity. Tie drumsticks together with kitchen string and tuck wing tips under.

4 Roast 20 minutes. *Reduce oven temperature to 375°F.* Roast 45 to 55 minutes or until chicken is cooked through (165°F), basting once with pan juices during last 10 minutes of cooking time. Remove chicken to cutting board; tent with foil. Let stand at least 15 minutes before carving. Garnish with parsley and lemon wedges.

1 whole chicken (about 4 pounds)

3 tablespoons butter, softened

1½ teaspoons salt

1 teaspoon onion powder

1 teaspoon dried thyme

½ teaspoon garlic powder

½ teaspoon paprika

½ teaspoon black pepper

Fresh parsley sprigs and lemon wedges (optional)

Nutrients Per Serving (¼ of total recipe)

CALORIES 360 **TOTAL FAT** 20g **CARBS** 1g **NET CARBS** 1g
DIETARY FIBER 0g **PROTEIN** 43g

Chicken Adobo

MAKES 6 SERVINGS

½ cup cider vinegar

½ cup reduced-sodium soy sauce

4 cloves garlic, minced

3 bay leaves

1 teaspoon black pepper

2½ pounds bone-in skin-on chicken thighs (about 6)

Sliced green onion (optional)

1 Combine vinegar, soy sauce, garlic, bay leaves and pepper in large saucepan or deep skillet; mix well. Add chicken; turn to coat. Arrange chicken skin side down in liquid.

2 Bring to a boil over high heat. Reduce heat to low; cover and simmer 30 minutes. Turn chicken skin side up. Cook, uncovered, 20 minutes. Preheat broiler. Line small baking sheet with foil.

3 Transfer chicken to prepared baking sheet, skin side up. Broil about 6 minutes or until skin is browned and crisp. Meanwhile, cook liquid in saucepan over high heat about 10 minutes or until reduced and slightly thickened.

4 Serve sauce over chicken. Garnish with green onion.

Nutrients Per Serving (⅙ of total recipe)

CALORIES 370 **TOTAL FAT** 27g **CARBS** 3g **NET CARBS** 3g
DIETARY FIBER 0g **PROTEIN** 28g

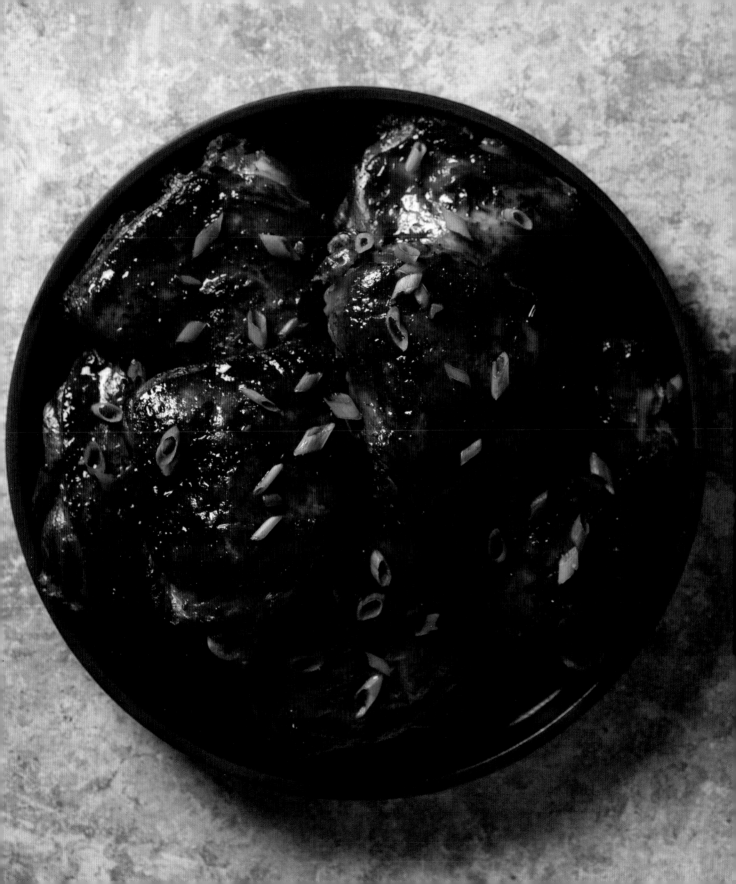

1 tablespoon chili powder

1 teaspoon paprika

1 teaspoon ground cumin

½ teaspoon dried oregano

½ teaspoon salt

¼ teaspoon garlic powder

¼ teaspoon onion powder

1 pound ground turkey

¾ cup water

1 bag (10 ounces) frozen riced cauliflower

2 cups shredded red cabbage

2 green onions, finely chopped

1 avocado, thinly sliced

2 plum tomatoes, diced

Minced fresh cilantro, sour cream and crumbled cotija cheese

Turkey Taco Bowls

MAKES 4 SERVINGS

1 Combine chili powder, paprika, cumin, oregano, salt, garlic powder and onion powder in small bowl.

2 Cook turkey in large nonstick skillet over medium-high heat 6 to 8 minutes or until no longer pink, stirring to break up meat. Stir in spice mix and water; bring to a boil. Reduce heat to medium-low; simmer 5 minutes, stirring occasionally. Set aside.

3 Heat cauliflower rice according to package directions. Divide among four bowls. Add turkey, cabbage, green onions, avocado and tomatoes. Serve with cilantro, sour cream and cotija cheese.

Nutrients Per Serving (¼ of total recipe)

CALORIES 250   **TOTAL FAT** 9g   **CARBS** 15g   **NET CARBS** 8g
DIETARY FIBER 7g   **PROTEIN** 31g

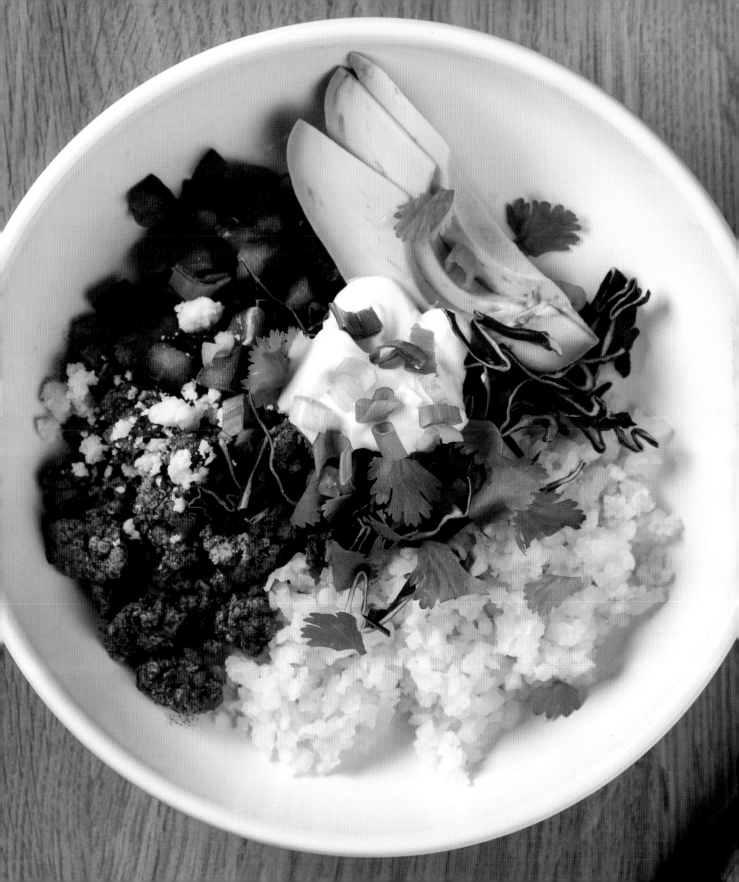

3 teaspoons olive oil, divided

1 cup coarsely chopped mushrooms

2 cups thinly sliced kale

1 tablespoon fresh lemon juice

½ teaspoon salt, divided

4 boneless skinless chicken breasts (about 4 ounces each)

¼ cup crumbled feta cheese

¼ teaspoon black pepper

Kale and Mushroom Stuffed Chicken Breasts

MAKES 4 SERVINGS

1 Heat 1 teaspoon oil in large skillet over medium-high heat. Add mushrooms; cook and stir 5 minutes or until mushrooms begin to brown. Add kale; cook and stir 8 minutes or until wilted. Sprinkle with lemon juice and ¼ teaspoon salt. Remove to small bowl. Let stand 5 to 10 minutes to cool slightly.

2 Meanwhile, place each chicken breast between sheets of plastic wrap. Pound with meat mallet or rolling pin to about ½-inch thickness.

3 Gently stir cheese into mushroom and kale mixture. Spoon ¼ cup mixture down center of each chicken breast. Roll up to enclose filling; secure with toothpicks. Sprinkle with remaining ¼ teaspoon salt and pepper.

4 Wipe out same skillet with paper towels. Add remaining 2 teaspoons oil to skillet; heat over medium heat. Add chicken; brown on all sides. Cover and cook 5 minutes per side or until no longer pink and chicken is cooked through (165°F). Remove toothpicks before serving.

Nutrients Per Serving (1 stuffed chicken breast)

CALORIES 192 **TOTAL FAT** 7g **CARBS** 4g **NET CARBS** 3g
DIETARY FIBER 1g **PROTEIN** 29g

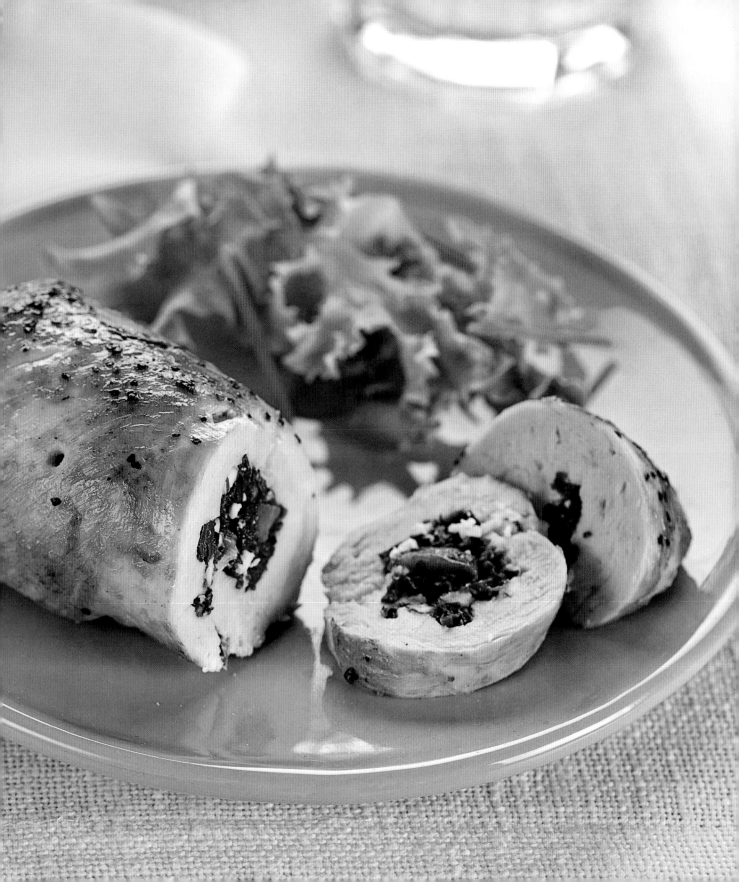

Chicken Skewers with Yogurt-Tahini Sauce

MAKES 8 SERVINGS

1 cup plain nonfat or regular Greek yogurt

¼ cup chopped fresh parsley, plus additional for garnish

¼ cup tahini

2 tablespoons lemon juice

1 clove garlic

¾ teaspoon salt, divided

1 tablespoon vegetable oil

2 teaspoons garam masala

1 pound boneless skinless chicken breasts, cut into 1-inch pieces

1 Spray grid with nonstick cooking spray. Prepare grill for direct cooking.

2 For sauce, combine yogurt, ¼ cup parsley, tahini, lemon juice, garlic and ¼ teaspoon salt in food processor or blender; process until smooth. Set aside.

3 Combine oil, garam masala and remaining ½ teaspoon salt in medium bowl. Add chicken; toss to coat. Thread chicken on eight 6-inch wooden or metal skewers.

4 Grill skewers over medium-high heat 5 minutes per side or until chicken is no longer pink and cooked through (165°F). Serve with sauce. Garnish with additional parsley.

Nutrients Per Serving
(1 skewer and about 2 tablespoons sauce)

CALORIES 145   **TOTAL FAT** 7g   **CARBS** 4g   **NET CARBS** 4g
DIETARY FIBER 0g   **PROTEIN** 16g

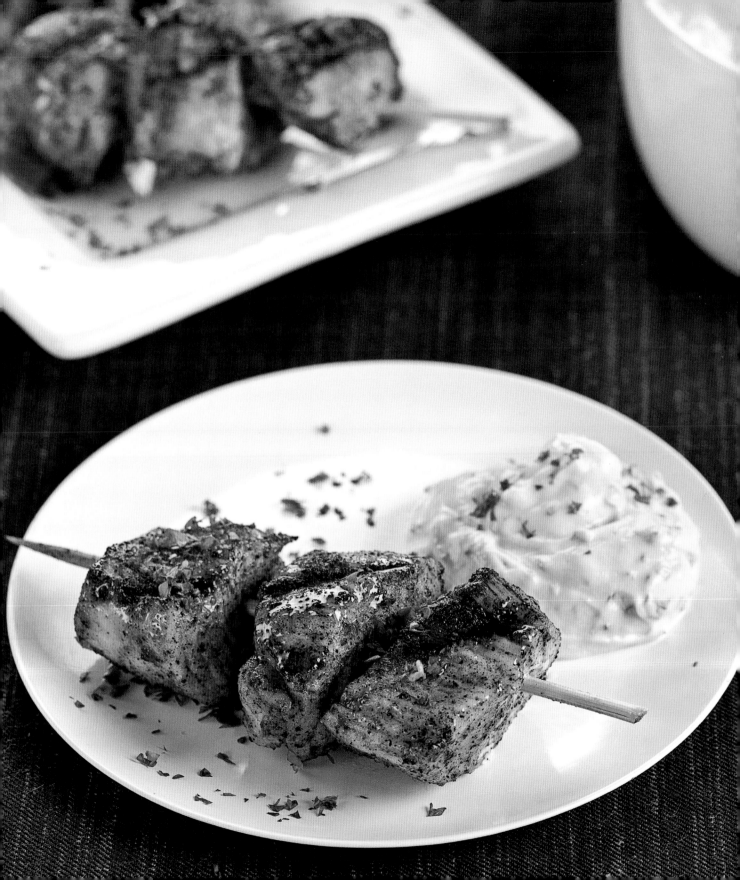

1 pound ground turkey

⅓ cup prepared pesto

⅓ cup grated Parmesan cheese, plus additional for garnish

¼ cup almond flour

1 egg

2 green onions, finely chopped

½ teaspoon salt, divided

2 tablespoons olive oil

2 cloves garlic, minced

⅛ teaspoon red pepper flakes

1 can (28 ounces) whole tomatoes, undrained, crushed with hands or coarsely chopped

1 tablespoon tomato paste

Zucchini noodles (optional)

Pesto Turkey Meatballs
MAKES 4 SERVINGS

1 Combine turkey, pesto, ⅓ cup cheese, almond flour, egg, green onions and ¼ teaspoon salt in medium bowl; mix well. Shape mixture into 24 balls (about 1¼ inches). Refrigerate meatballs while preparing sauce.

2 Heat oil in large saucepan or Dutch oven over medium heat. Add garlic and red pepper flakes; cook and stir 2 minutes. Add tomatoes with liquid, tomato paste and remaining ¼ teaspoon salt; cook 5 minutes or until sauce begins to simmer, stirring occasionally.

3 Remove about 1 cup sauce from saucepan. Arrange meatballs in single layer in saucepan; pour reserved sauce over meatballs. Reduce heat to medium-low; cover and cook 20 minutes.

4 Uncover; increase heat to medium-high. Cook about 10 minutes or until sauce thickens slightly and meatballs are cooked through. Serve over zucchini noodles, if desired, and garnish with additional cheese.

Nutrients Per Serving (6 meatballs and ¼ of sauce)
CALORIES 390 **TOTAL FAT** 23g **CARBS** 12g **NET CARBS** 8g
DIETARY FIBER 4g **PROTEIN** 37g

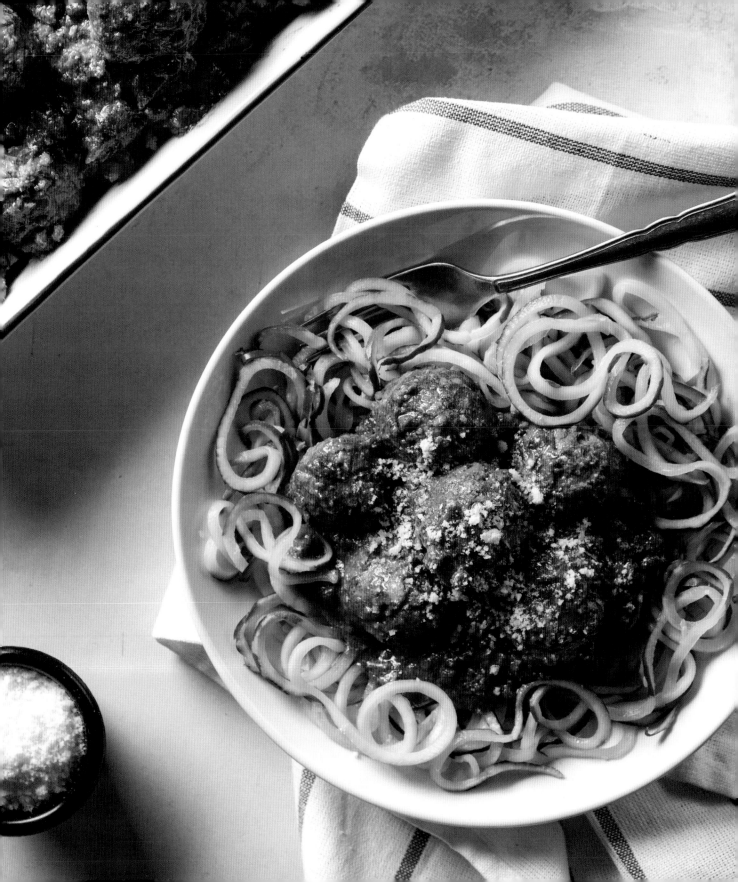

1 cut-up whole chicken (about 3 to 4 pounds)

1 tablespoon olive oil

2 teaspoons Greek seasoning

1 teaspoon salt

1 teaspoon black pepper

Juice of 1 lemon

Lemony Greek Chicken

MAKES 4 SERVINGS

1 Preheat oven to 400°F.

2 Brush chicken with oil. Arrange on two large baking dishes, skin side up. Combine Greek seasoning, salt and pepper in small bowl; sprinkle half over chicken. Bake 30 minutes.

3 Turn chicken pieces over. Sprinkle with remaining seasoning mixture and lemon juice. Bake 30 minutes or until chicken is cooked through (165°F).

Nutrients Per Serving (¼ of total recipe)

CALORIES 240   **TOTAL FAT** 12g   **CARBS** 0g   **NET CARBS** 0g
DIETARY FIBER 0g   **PROTEIN** 32g

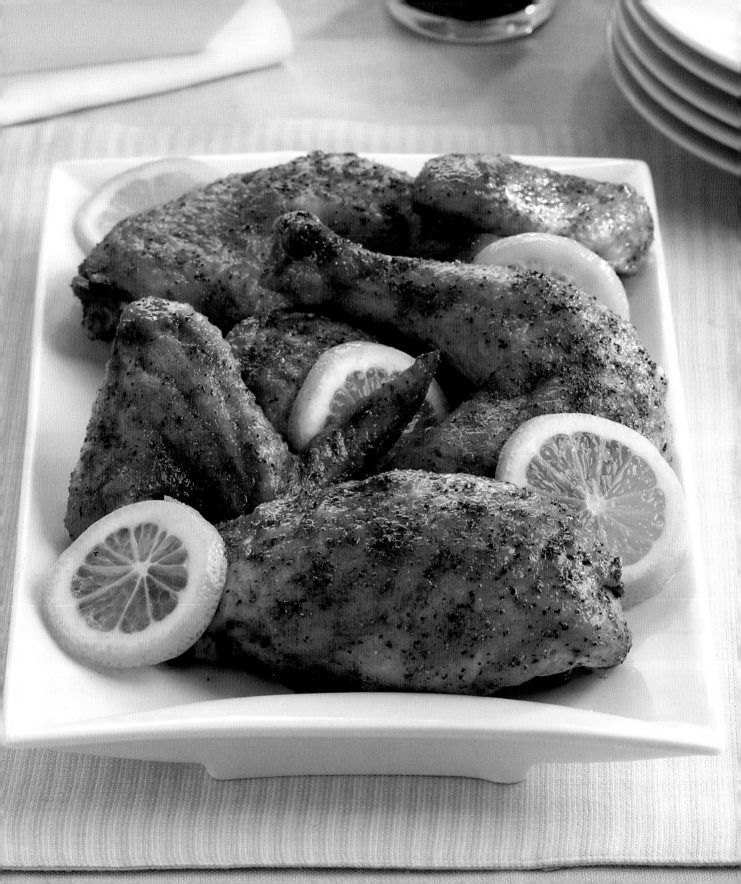

Turkey and Veggie Meatballs with Fennel

MAKES 6 SERVINGS

½ cup finely chopped green onions

½ cup finely chopped green bell pepper

⅓ cup almond flour

2 egg whites

2 tablespoons whipping cream

¼ cup shredded carrot

¼ cup grated Parmesan cheese

2 cloves garlic, minced

½ teaspoon Italian seasoning

¼ teaspoon fennel seeds

¼ teaspoon salt

⅛ teaspoon red pepper flakes (optional)

1 pound ground turkey

1 teaspoon extra virgin olive oil

1 Combine green onions, bell pepper, almond flour, egg whites, cream, carrot, cheese, garlic, Italian seasoning, fennel, salt and red pepper flakes, if desired, in large bowl. Add turkey; mix well. Shape into 36 (1-inch) balls.

2 Heat oil in large nonstick skillet over medium-high heat. Add meatballs; cook 10 to 12 minutes or until no longer pink in center, turning frequently. Serve immediately or cool and freeze.*

*To freeze, cool completely and place in gallon-size resealable food storage bag. Release any excess air from bag and seal. Freeze bag flat for easier storage and faster thawing. To reheat, place meatballs in a 12×8-inch microwavable dish and cook on HIGH 20 to 30 seconds or until hot.

Nutrients Per Serving (6 meatballs)

CALORIES 170   **TOTAL FAT** 8g   **CARBS** 3g   **NET CARBS** 2g
DIETARY FIBER 1g   **PROTEIN** 23g

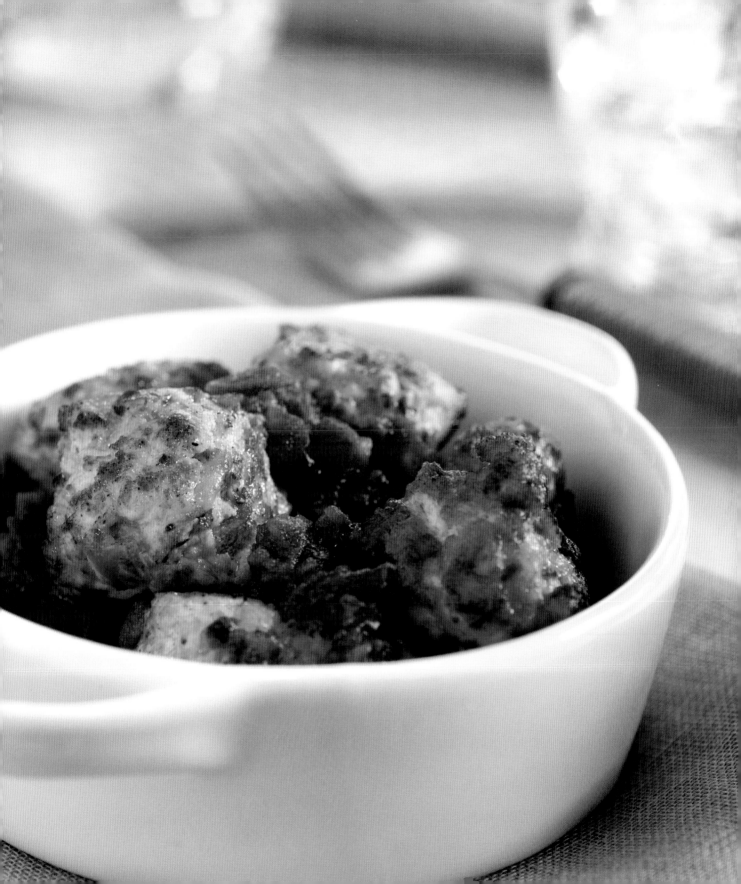

2 cloves garlic

1 cup packed fresh
   cilantro leaves

1 tablespoon plus
   2 teaspoons soy
   sauce, divided

1 tablespoon peanut or
   vegetable oil

4 boneless chicken
   breasts (about
   1¼ pounds)

1 tablespoon dark
   sesame oil

Cilantro-Stuffed Chicken Breasts
MAKES 4 SERVINGS

1 Preheat oven to 350°F. Mince garlic in blender or food processor. Add cilantro; process until cilantro is minced. Add 2 teaspoons soy sauce and peanut oil; process until paste forms.

2 With rubber spatula or fingers, spread about 1 tablespoon cilantro mixture evenly under skin of each chicken breast, taking care not to puncture skin.

3 Line baking pan with foil; place rack in pan. Place chicken on rack. Combine remaining 1 tablespoon soy sauce and sesame oil in small bowl. Brush half of mixture evenly over chicken.

4 Bake 25 minutes; brush remaining soy sauce mixture evenly over chicken. Bake 10 minutes or until juices run clear and chicken is cooked through (165°F).

Nutrients Per Serving (1 stuffed chicken breast)
CALORIES 180   **TOTAL FAT** 9g   **CARBS** 1g   **NET CARBS** 1g
DIETARY FIBER 0g   **PROTEIN** 21g

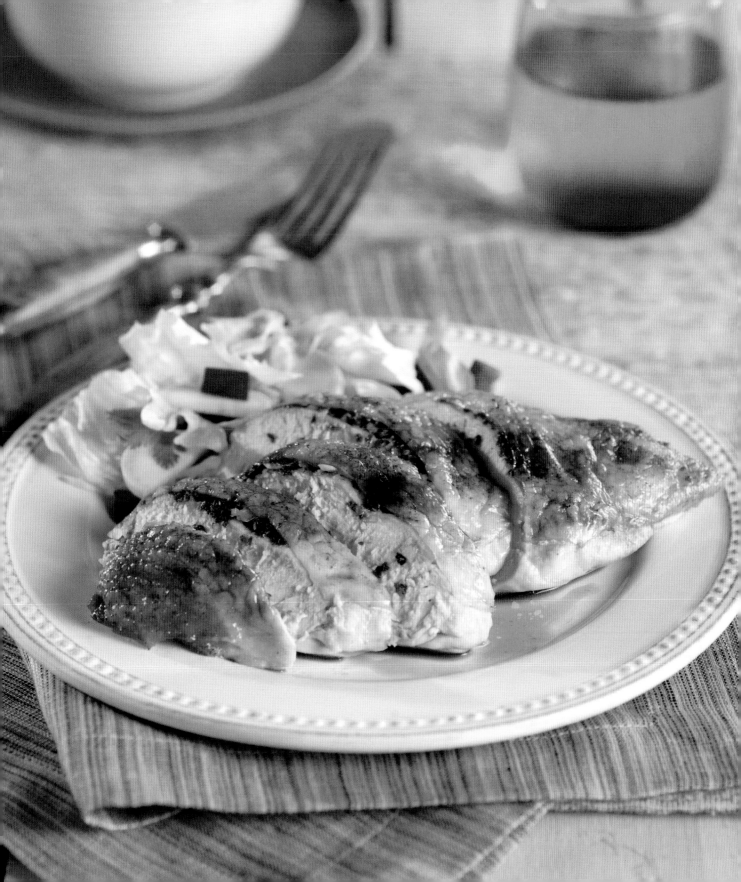

Greek-Style Chicken Wings with Tzatziki Sauce

MAKES 8 SERVINGS

Chicken Wings

2 tablespoons olive oil, divided

5 pounds chicken wings, tips removed and split at joints

2 teaspoons dried oregano

½ teaspoon salt

¼ teaspoon black pepper

2 tablespoons fresh lemon juice

Tzatziki Sauce

1 medium cucumber

2 cups plain Greek yogurt

2 tablespoons fresh lemon juice

2 tablespoons olive oil

1 clove garlic, minced

½ teaspoon salt

1 Preheat oven to 375°F. Grease large rimmed baking sheet with 1 tablespoon oil. Combine chicken, remaining 1 tablespoon oil, oregano, ½ teaspoon salt and pepper in large bowl; toss until well coated. Arrange on prepared baking sheet.

2 Bake 45 to 60 minutes or until wings are cooked through, well browned and crisp. Drizzle with 2 tablespoons lemon juice.

3 Meanwhile for tzatziki sauce, peel cucumber and slice in half lengthwise. Scoop seeds from both halves of cucumber. Coarsely grate cucumber into medium bowl. Stir in yogurt, 2 tablespoons lemon juice, 2 tablespoons olive oil and garlic; season with ½ teaspoon salt. Cover and refrigerate until ready to use. Serve with wings.

Nutrients Per Serving (⅛ of total recipe)

CALORIES 660   **TOTAL FAT** 46g   **CARBS** 4g   **NET CARBS** 3g
DIETARY FIBER 1g   **PROTEIN** 55g

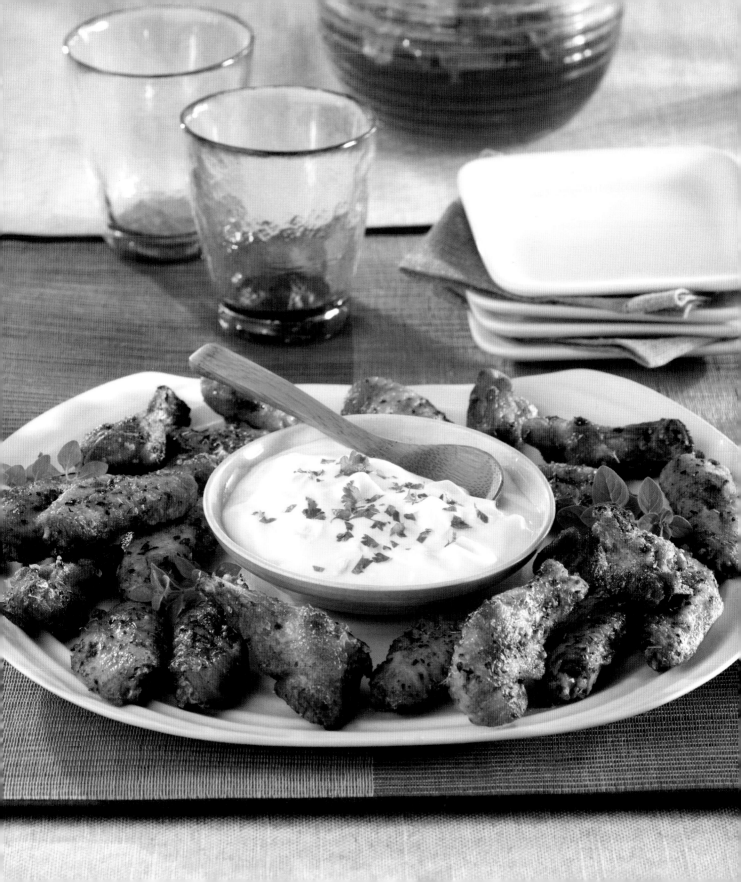

3 tablespoons extra
   virgin olive oil,
   divided
1 pound spicy Italian
   sausage, cut into
   1-inch pieces
1 whole chicken (about
   3 pounds), cut into
   10 pieces*
1 teaspoon salt, divided
1 large onion, chopped
2 red, yellow or orange
   bell peppers, cut
   into ¼-inch strips
3 cloves garlic, minced
½ cup dry white wine
   (such as sauvignon
   blanc)
½ cup chicken broth
½ cup coarsely chopped
   seeded hot cherry
   peppers
½ cup liquid from cherry
   pepper jar
1 teaspoon dried
   oregano
   Additional salt and
   black pepper
¼ cup chopped fresh
   Italian parsley

*Or purchase 2 bone-in
chicken leg quarters and
2 chicken breasts; separate
drumsticks and thighs and
cut breasts in half.

Chicken Scarpiello
MAKES 6 SERVINGS

1 Heat 1 tablespoon oil in large skillet over medium-high heat. Add sausage; cook about 10 minutes or until well browned on all sides, stirring occasionally. Remove sausage from skillet; set aside.

2 Heat 1 tablespoon oil in same skillet. Sprinkle chicken with ½ teaspoon salt; arrange skin side down in single layer in skillet (cook in batches, if necessary). Cook about 6 minutes per side or until browned. Remove chicken from skillet; set aside. Drain oil from skillet.

3 Heat remaining 1 tablespoon oil in skillet. Add onion and ½ teaspoon salt; cook and stir 2 minutes or until onion is softened, scraping up browned bits from bottom of skillet. Add bell peppers and garlic; cook and stir 5 minutes. Stir in wine; cook until liquid is reduced by half. Stir in broth, cherry peppers, cherry pepper liquid and oregano. Season with additional salt and black pepper; bring to a simmer.

4 Return sausage and chicken along with any accumulated juices to skillet. Partially cover skillet; simmer 10 minutes. Uncover; simmer 15 minutes or until chicken is cooked through (165°F). Sprinkle with parsley.

Tip: If too much liquid remains in the skillet when the chicken is cooked through, remove the chicken and sausage and continue simmering the sauce to reduce it slightly.

Nutrients Per Serving (⅙ of total recipe)

CALORIES 500   **TOTAL FAT** 35g   **CARBS** 11g   **NET CARBS** 10g
DIETARY FIBER 1g   **PROTEIN** 30g

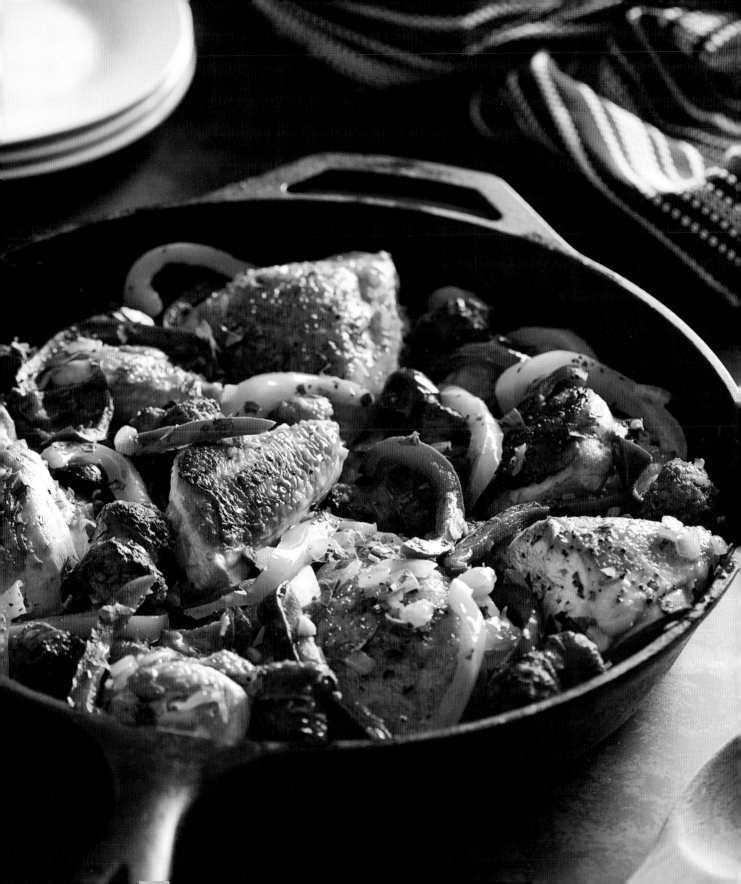

Greek Chicken Burgers with Cucumber Yogurt Sauce

MAKES 4 SERVINGS

½ cup plus 2 tablespoons plain nonfat or whole-milk Greek yogurt

½ medium cucumber, peeled, seeded and finely chopped

Juice of ½ lemon

3 cloves garlic, minced, divided

2 teaspoons finely chopped fresh mint *or* ½ teaspoon dried mint

⅛ teaspoon salt

⅛ teaspoon ground white pepper

1 pound ground chicken

3 ounces crumbled feta cheese

4 large kalamata olives, rinsed, patted dry and minced

1 egg

½ to 1 teaspoon dried oregano

¼ teaspoon black pepper

Mixed baby lettuce (optional)

1 Combine yogurt, cucumber, lemon juice, 2 cloves garlic, mint, salt and white pepper in medium bowl; mix well. Cover and refrigerate until ready to serve.

2 Combine chicken, cheese, olives, egg, oregano, black pepper and remaining 1 clove garlic in large bowl; mix well. Shape mixture into four patties.

3 Spray grill pan with nonstick cooking spray; heat over medium-high heat. Grill patties 5 to 7 minutes per side or until cooked through (165°F).

4 Serve burgers with sauce and mixed greens, if desired.

Nutrients Per Serving (1 burger and ¼ of sauce)

CALORIES 260   **TOTAL FAT** 14g   **CARBS** 4g   **NET CARBS** 3g
DIETARY FIBER 1g   **PROTEIN** 29g

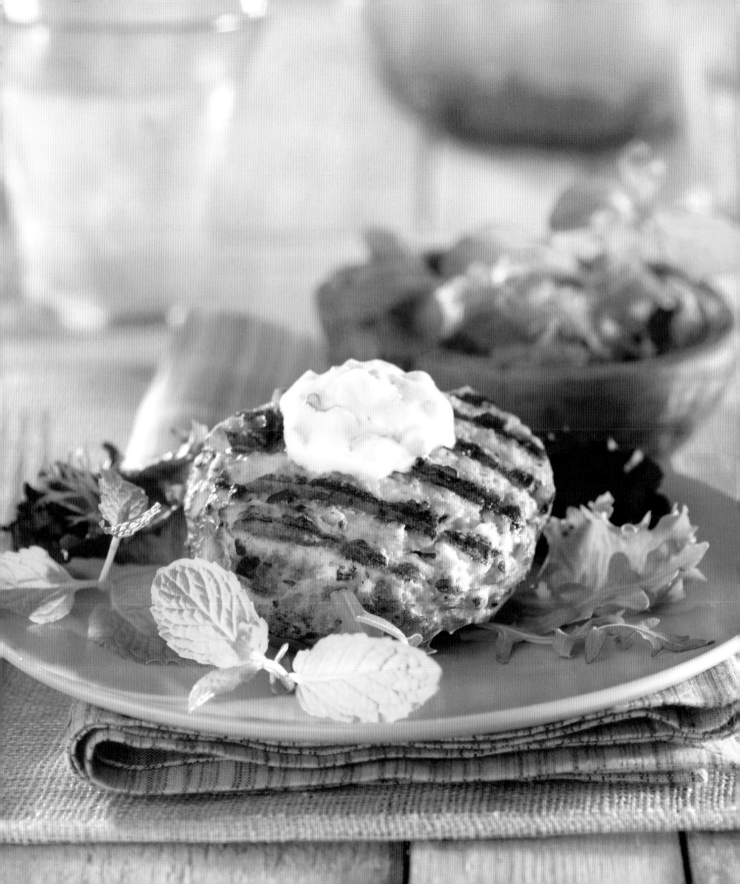

1 roasting chicken or
   capon (about
   6½ pounds)
1 tablespoon peanut
   or vegetable oil
2 cloves garlic, minced
1 tablespoon soy sauce

Crispy Roasted Chicken
MAKES 8 SERVINGS

1 Preheat oven to 350°F. Place chicken on rack in shallow, foil-lined roasting pan.

2 Combine oil and garlic in small cup; brush evenly over chicken. Roast 15 to 20 minutes per pound (about 90 minutes for a 6-pound chicken) or until internal temperature reaches 170°F when tested with meat thermometer inserted into thickest part of thigh not touching bone.

3 *Increase oven temperature to 450°F.* Remove drippings from pan; discard. Brush chicken evenly with soy sauce. Roast 5 to 10 minutes or until skin is very crisp and deep golden brown. Transfer chicken to cutting board; let stand 10 to 15 minutes before carving. Internal temperature will continue to rise 5° to 10°F during stand time. Cover and refrigerate leftovers up to 3 days or freeze up to 3 months.

Nutrients Per Serving (⅛ **of chicken)**

CALORIES 597   **TOTAL FAT** 42g   **CARBS** 1g   **NET CARBS** 0g
DIETARY FIBER 1g   **PROTEIN** 50g

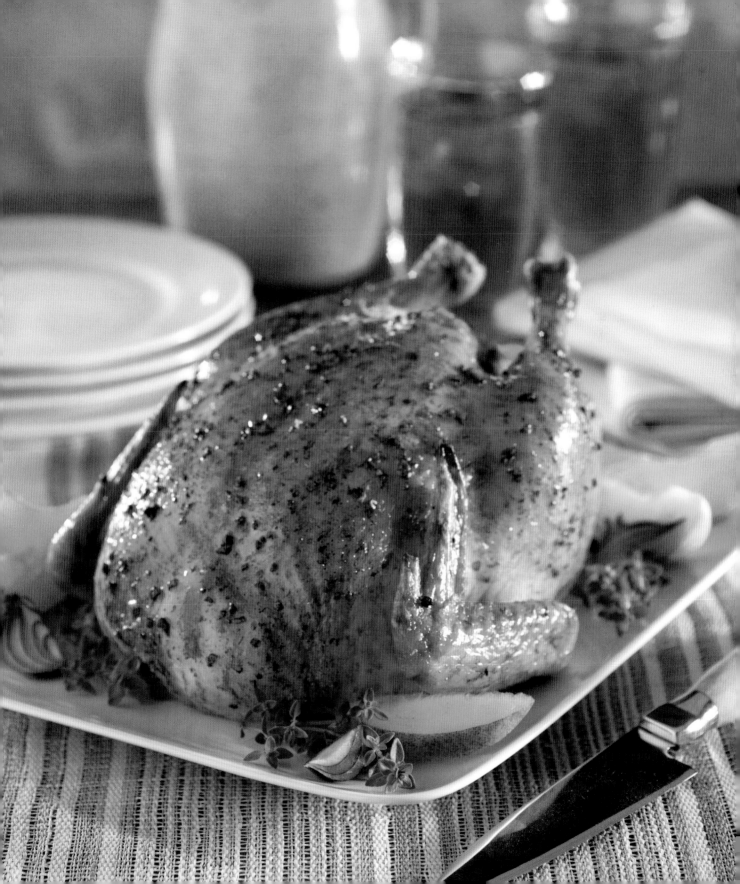

Chicken Piccata

MAKES 4 SERVINGS

3 tablespoons almond flour

½ teaspoon salt

¼ teaspoon black pepper

4 boneless skinless chicken breasts (4 ounces each)

2 teaspoons olive oil

1 teaspoon butter

2 cloves garlic, minced

¾ cup chicken broth

1 tablespoon fresh lemon juice

2 tablespoons chopped fresh Italian parsley

1 tablespoon capers, drained

1 Combine almond flour, salt and pepper in shallow dish. Reserve 1 tablespoon flour mixture; set aside.

2 Pound chicken between waxed paper to ½-inch thickness with flat side of meat mallet or rolling pin. Coat chicken with remaining flour mixture, shaking off excess.

3 Heat oil and butter in large nonstick skillet over medium heat. Add chicken; cook 4 to 5 minutes per side or until no longer pink in center and cooked through (165°F). Transfer to serving platter; cover loosely with foil.

4 Add garlic to same skillet; cook and stir 1 minute. Add reserved flour mixture; cook and stir 1 minute. Add broth and lemon juice; cook 2 minutes or until thickened, stirring frequently. Stir in parsley and capers; spoon sauce over chicken.

Nutrients Per Serving
(1 chicken breast and ¼ cup of sauce)

CALORIES 180   **TOTAL FAT** 7g   **CARBS** 2g   **NET CARBS** 1g
DIETARY FIBER 1g   **PROTEIN** 27g

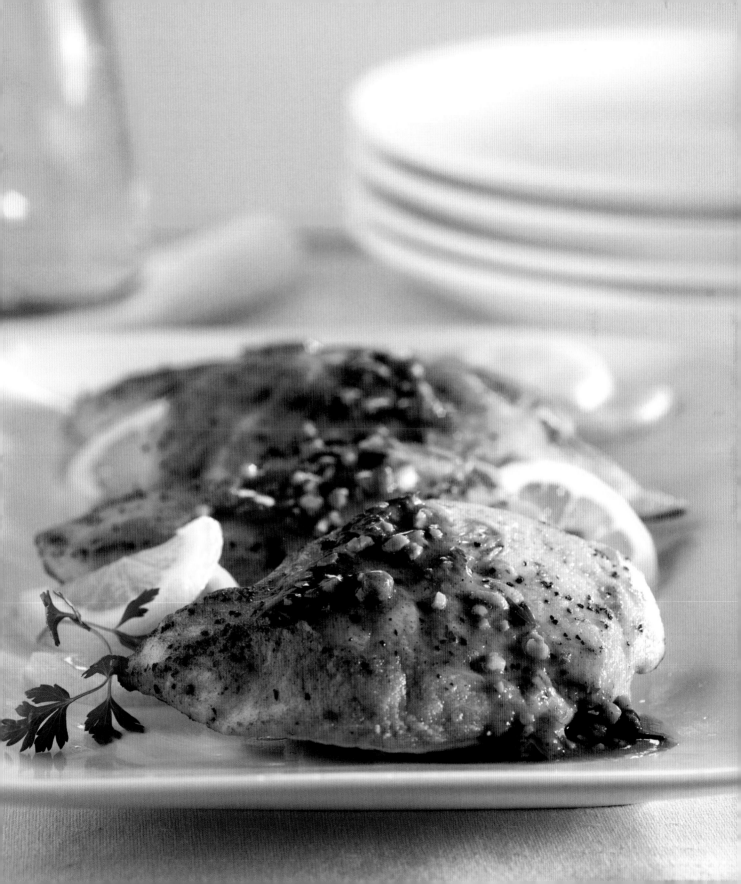

- 1 tablespoon canola oil
- 1 red bell pepper, chopped
- 1 pound boneless skinless chicken thighs, trimmed and cut into 1-inch pieces
- 1 package (12 ounces) Cajun andouille or spicy chicken sausage, sliced ½ inch thick
- ½ cup chicken broth
- 1 can (28 ounces) crushed tomatoes with roasted garlic
- ¼ cup finely chopped green onions
- 1 bay leaf
- ½ teaspoon dried basil
- ½ teaspoon black pepper
- ¼ to ½ teaspoon red pepper flakes
- 6 lemon wedges (optional)

Sausage and Chicken Gumbo

MAKES 6 SERVINGS

1 Heat oil in large saucepan over medium-high heat. Add bell pepper; cook and stir 2 to 3 minutes. Add chicken; cook and stir about 2 minutes or until browned. Add sausage; cook and stir 2 minutes or until browned. Add broth; scrape up browned bits from bottom of saucepan.

2 Add tomatoes, green onions, bay leaf, basil, black pepper and red pepper flakes; simmer 15 minutes. Remove and discard bay leaf. Garnish each serving with lemon wedge.

Nutrients Per Serving (1⅓ cups)

CALORIES 239 **TOTAL FAT** 11g **CARBS** 10g **NET CARBS** 8g
DIETARY FIBER 2g **PROTEIN** 28g

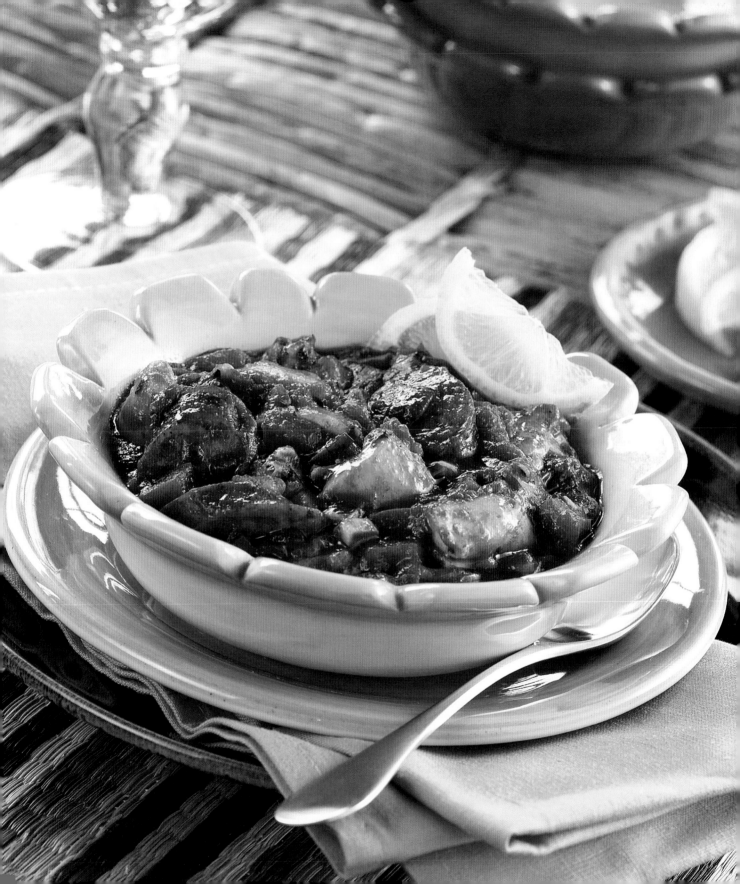

Chicken

- 1 tablespoon olive oil
- 1 teaspoon salt
- 1 teaspoon dried oregano
- 1 teaspoon paprika
- ½ teaspoon black pepper
- 1 clove garlic, minced
- 2 boneless skinless chicken breasts (8 ounces each)

Salad and Dressing

- ¼ cup mayonnaise
- 1 tablespoon olive oil
- 1 tablespoon Dijon mustard
- 1 clove garlic, minced
- ⅛ teaspoon Italian seasoning, dried basil or dried oregano
- Salt and black pepper
- 4 cups packed baby spinach
- 1 avocado, halved and sliced
- 1 cup cherry tomatoes, quartered
- ¼ white onion, very thinly sliced (optional)
- Black sesame seeds (optional)

Grilled Chicken with Avocado and Spinach
MAKES 2 SERVINGS

1 Oil grid. Prepare grill for direct cooking.*

2 Combine 1 tablespoon oil, salt, oregano, paprika, black pepper and 1 clove garlic in large bowl. Rub mixture all over chicken.

3 Grill chicken over medium-high heat about 5 minutes per side or until no longer pink in center and cooked through (165°F).* Remove to cutting board; let stand 5 minutes before slicing.

4 For sauce, whisk mayonnaise, 1 tablespoon oil, mustard, 1 clove garlic and Italian seasoning in small bowl. Season to taste with salt and black pepper.

5 Divide spinach between two serving bowls. Top with chicken, avocados, tomatoes, onion and sesame seeds, if desired.

Or use stovetop grill pan; cook chicken in 1 tablespoon of olive oil over medium-high heat about 10 minutes or until chicken is cooked through, turning once.

Nutrients Per Serving (½ of total recipe)

CALORIES 790   **TOTAL FAT** 54g   **CARBS** 17g   **NET CARBS** 6g
DIETARY FIBER 11g   **PROTEIN** 57g

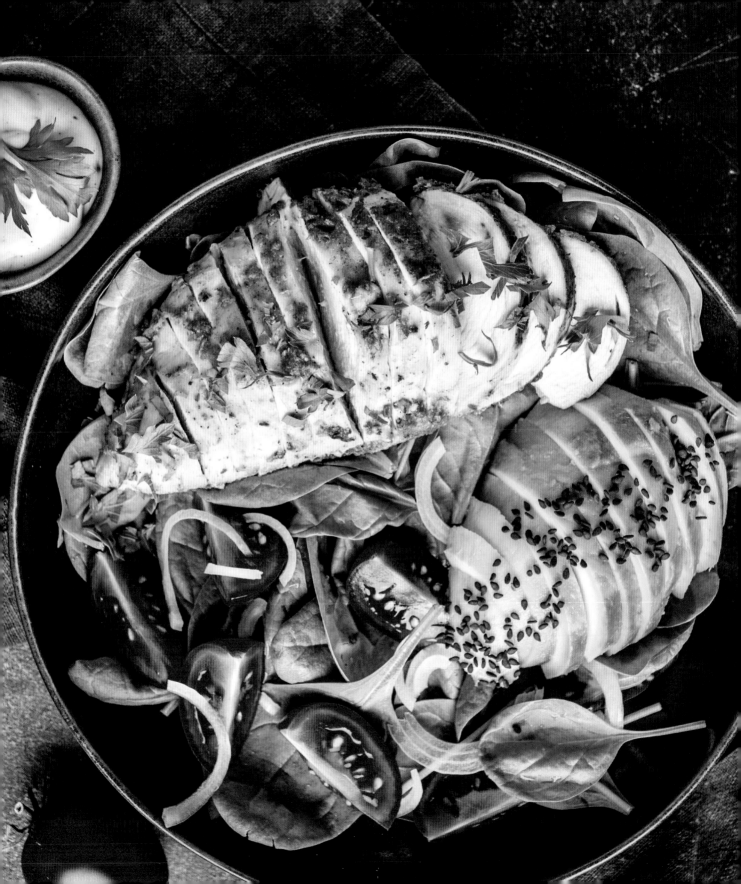

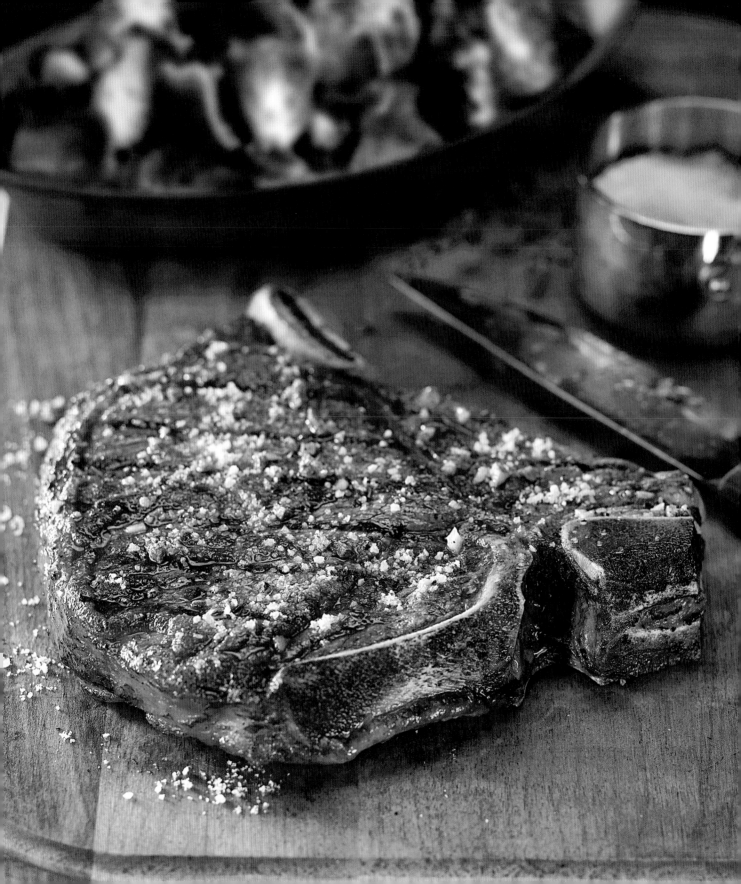

Beef and Pork

Steak Parmesan
MAKES 2 SERVINGS

1 Prepare grill for direct cooking. Combine garlic, oil, salt and pepper in small bowl; rub all over both sides of steaks. Let stand 15 minutes.

2 Place steaks on grid over medium-high heat. Cover; grill 14 to 19 minutes or until internal temperature reaches 145°F for medium-rare doneness, turning once.

3 Transfer steaks to cutting board; sprinkle with cheese. Tent with foil; let stand 5 minutes. Serve immediately.

Tip: For a smoky flavor, soak 2 cups hickory or oak wood chips in cold water to cover at least 30 minutes. Drain and scatter over hot coals before grilling.

4 cloves garlic, minced
1 tablespoon olive oil
1 tablespoon coarse salt
1 teaspoon black pepper
2 beef T-bone or Porterhouse steaks, cut 1 to 1¼ inch thick (about 2 pounds)
¼ cup grated Parmesan cheese

Nutrients Per Serving (½ of total recipe)
CALORIES 390 **TOTAL FAT** 27g **CARBS** 2g **NET CARBS** 2g
DIETARY FIBER 0g **PROTEIN** 34g

3 tablespoons soy sauce

1½ teaspoons dark sesame oil

3 cloves garlic, minced, divided

12 ounces beef for stir-fry

1 seedless cucumber, thinly sliced

⅓ cup rice vinegar

¼ teaspoon plus ⅛ teaspoon salt, divided

2 tablespoons plus 1 teaspoon vegetable oil, divided

4 ounces shiitake mushrooms, stemmed and thinly sliced

3 cups fresh spinach

1 tablespoon water

3 cups frozen cauliflower rice, cooked according to package directions

1 carrot, julienned

4 eggs, cooked sunny side up or over easy

Gochujang sauce or sriracha sauce

Bibimbap with Cauliflower Rice
MAKES 4 SERVINGS

1 Combine 2 tablespoons soy sauce, sesame oil and 1 clove garlic in medium bowl. Add beef; stir to thoroughly coat with marinade. Refrigerate 30 minutes to 1 hour.

2 For cucumbers, combine cucumbers, vinegar and ⅛ teaspoon salt in large bowl. Let stand at room temperature until ready to serve.

3 For mushrooms, heat 1 tablespoon vegetable oil in medium skillet over high heat. Add mushrooms and remaining ¼ teaspoon salt; cook and stir 2 to 3 minutes or until mushrooms are browned and tender. Transfer mushrooms to medium bowl.

4 For spinach, heat 1 teaspoon vegetable oil in same skillet over high heat. Add spinach and 1 tablespoon water; cook until spinach is wilted. Add remaining 2 cloves garlic; cook 30 seconds or until garlic is lightly browned. Stir in remaining 1 tablespoon soy sauce. Transfer spinach to another medium bowl.

5 For beef, heat remaining 1 tablespoon vegetable oil in same skillet over high heat. Add beef and marinade; cook and stir 2 to 3 minutes or until beef is no longer pink.

6 For each serving, divide cauliflower rice among serving bowls. Top with cucumbers, carrots, spinach, mushrooms and beef. Top with egg and serve with desired sauce.

Nutrients Per Serving (¼ of total recipe)
CALORIES 367　**TOTAL FAT** 20g　**CARBS** 19g　**NET CARBS** 15g
DIETARY FIBER 4g　**PROTEIN** 20g

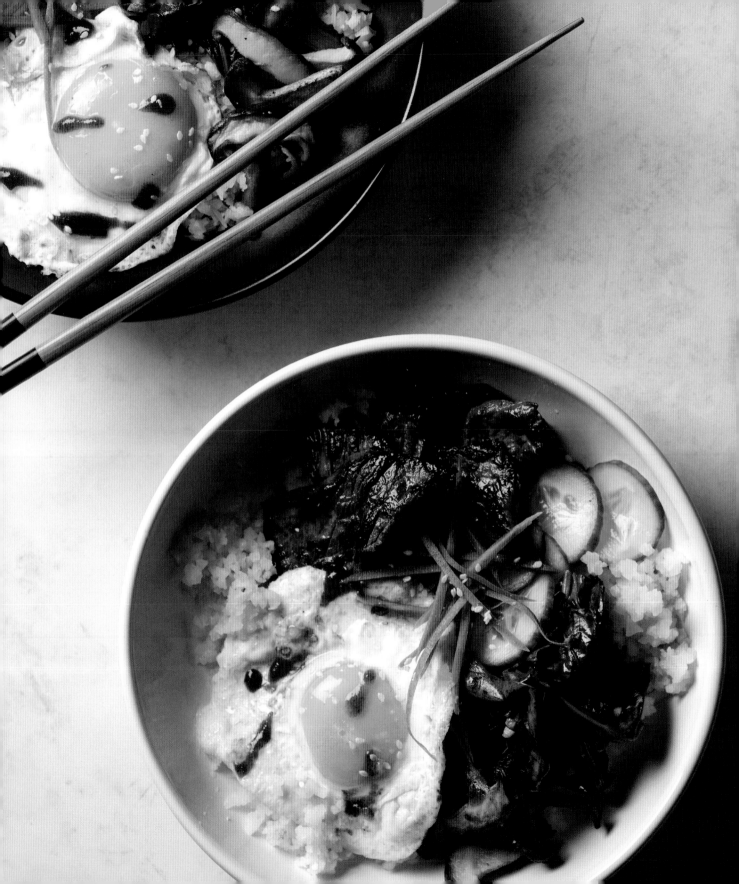

1 package (16 ounces) white mushrooms, stemmed and halved

3 tablespoons olive oil, divided

1 teaspoon salt, divided

1 head cauliflower, separated into florets and thinly sliced

¼ teaspoon chipotle chili powder

1 package (about 13 ounces) smoked sausage, cut into ¼-inch slices

1 tablespoon Dijon mustard

½ red onion, thinly sliced

6 ounces Gouda cheese, cubed

Cauliflower, Sausage and Gouda Sheet Pan
MAKES 6 SERVINGS

1 Preheat oven to 400°F.

2 Place mushrooms in medium bowl. Drizzle with 1 tablespoon oil and sprinkle with ½ teaspoon salt; toss to coat. Spread on sheet pan.

3 Place cauliflower, remaining 2 tablespoons oil, ½ teaspoon salt and chipotle chili powder in same bowl; toss to coat. Spread on sheet pan with mushrooms.

4 Combine sausage and mustard in same bowl; stir until well coated. Arrange sausage over vegetables; top with onion.

5 Roast 30 minutes. Remove from oven; place cheese cubes on top of cauliflower. Bake 5 minutes or until cheese is melted and cauliflower is tender.

Nutrients Per Serving (⅙ of total recipe)

CALORIES 340   **TOTAL FAT** 24g   **CARBS** 9g   **NET CARBS** 7g
DIETARY FIBER 2g   **PROTEIN** 20g

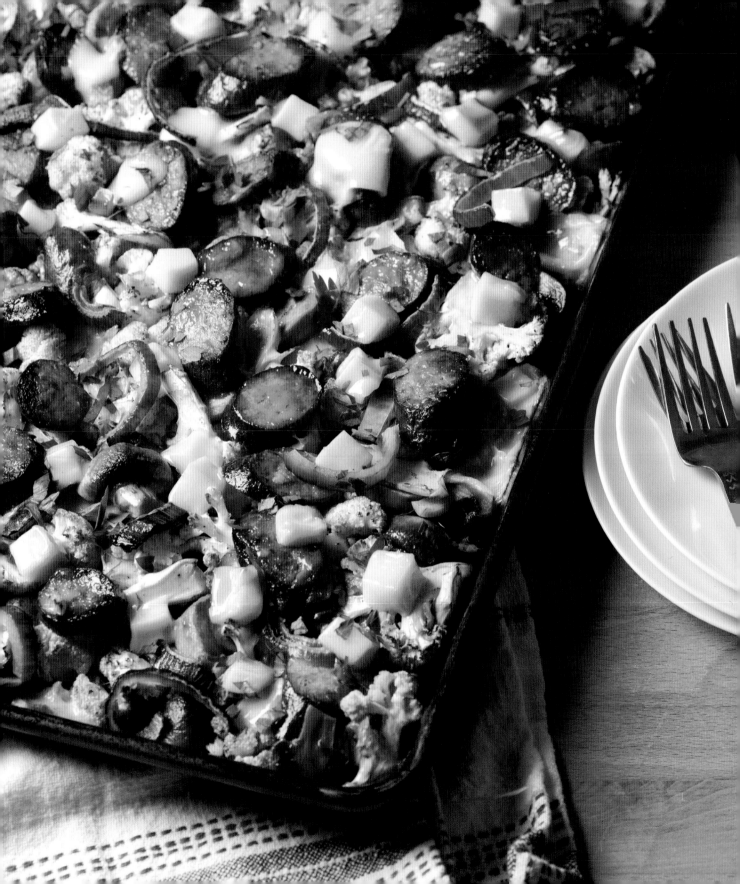

Bacon Smashburger
MAKES 4 SERVINGS

4 slices bacon, cut in
half

1 pound ground beef
Salt and black pepper

4 slices sharp Cheddar
cheese

4 eggs (optional)

1 Cook bacon in large skillet over medium-high heat until crisp. Remove from skillet; drain on paper towels. Drain all but 1 tablespoon fat from skillet.

2 Divide beef into four portions and shape lightly into loose balls. Place in same skillet over medium-high heat. Smash with spatula to flatten into thin patties; sprinkle with salt and pepper. Cook 2 to 3 minutes or until edges and bottoms are browned. Flip burgers and top with 1 slice of cheese. Cook 2 to 3 minutes for medium rare or to desired degree of doneness. Transfer to plates.

3 If desired, crack eggs into hot skillet. Cook over medium heat about 3 minutes or until whites are opaque and yolks are desired degree of doneness, flipping once, if desired, for overeasy. Place on burgers; top with bacon.

Nutrients Per Serving (1 burger without egg)
CALORIES 330   **TOTAL FAT** 23g   **CARBS** 0g   **NET CARBS** 0g
DIETARY FIBER 0g   **PROTEIN** 31g

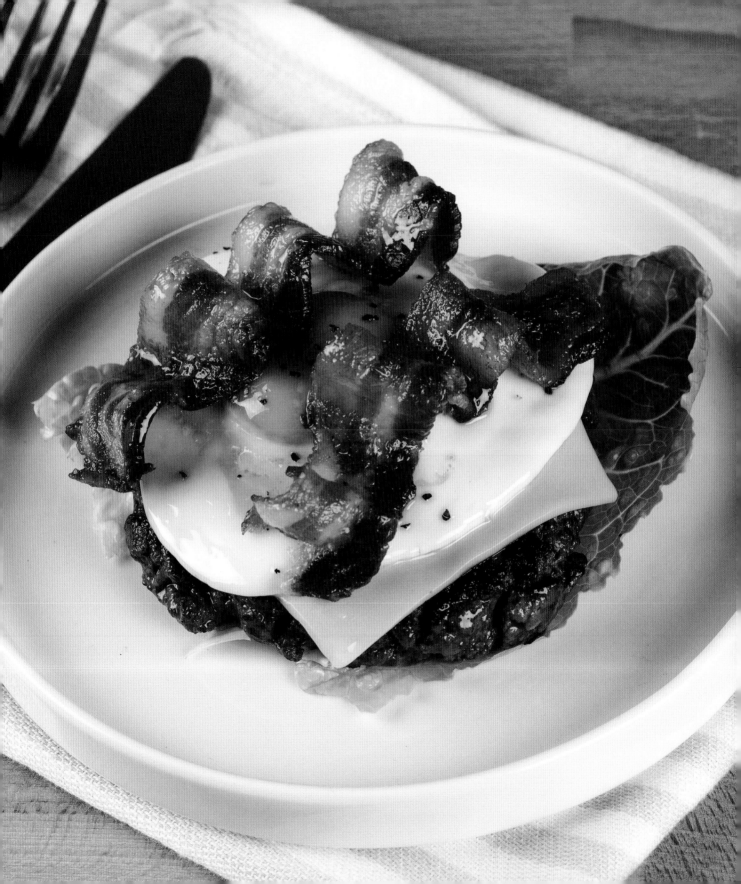

1 pork tenderloin (about 1 pound)

1 clove garlic, thinly sliced

1 teaspoon dried oregano

Grated peel of 1 lemon

1 cup plain yogurt

2 cups shredded red cabbage

½ cup chopped green onions (green parts only)

2 tablespoons balsamic vinegar

1 tablespoon canola oil

¾ teaspoon salt, divided

½ teaspoon black pepper, divided

Pork Tenderloin with Red Cabbage Slaw
MAKES 4 SERVINGS

1 Pierce pork in several places with knife tip. Insert garlic slice, pinch of oregano and pinch of lemon peel. Place pork in bowl. Add yogurt; spread over all sides of pork to coat. Cover; refrigerate 4 to 6 hours.

2 Meanwhile for slaw, combine cabbage, green onions, vinegar, oil, ¼ teaspoon salt and ¼ teaspoon pepper in medium bowl; refrigerate until ready to serve.

3 Preheat oven to 425°F. Remove pork from yogurt, scraping off any excess. Sprinkle pork with remaining ½ teaspoon salt and ¼ teaspoon pepper. Place pork on shallow rack over roasting pan.

4 Roast 35 to 40 minutes, turning over once, or until meat thermometer registers 145°F. Let rest 5 minutes. Slice ¼ inch thick on the diagonal; serve with slaw.

Nutrients Per Serving (3 ounces pork and ½ cup slaw)
CALORIES 222 **TOTAL FAT** 7g **CARBS** 11g **NET CARBS** 10g
DIETARY FIBER 1g **PROTEIN** 28g

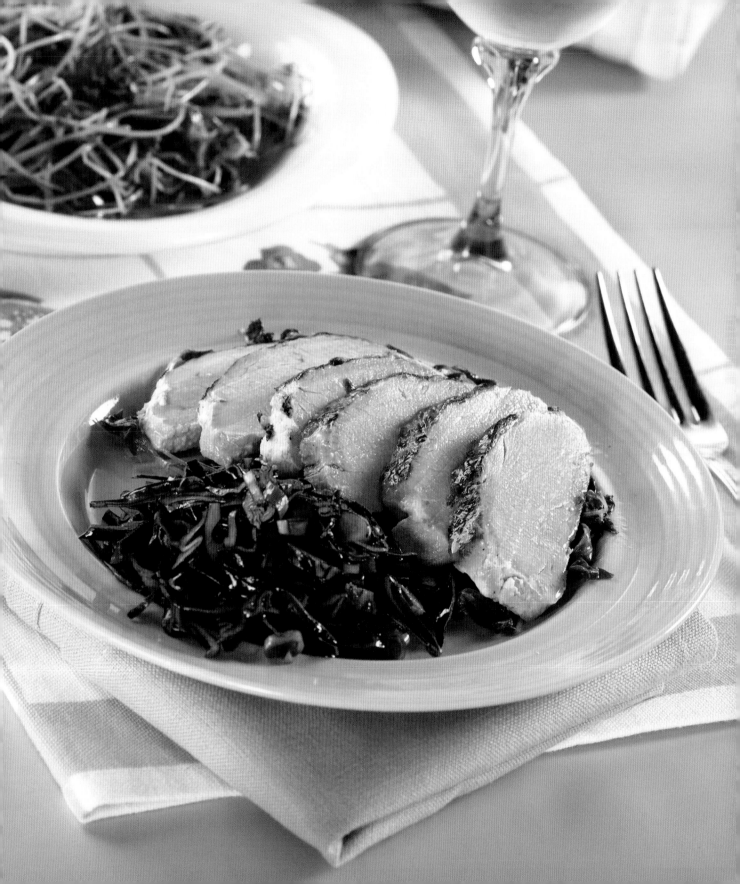

Balsamic Grilled Pork Chops

MAKES 2 SERVINGS

2 tablespoons balsamic vinegar

2 tablespoons soy sauce

1 teaspoon Dijon mustard

⅛ teaspoon red pepper flakes

2 boneless pork chops, trimmed of fat (8 ounces total)

1 Combine vinegar, soy sauce, mustard and red pepper flakes in small bowl. Stir until well blended. Reserve 1 tablespoon marinade; refrigerate until needed.

2 Place pork in large resealable food storage bag. Pour remaining marinade over pork. Seal bag; turn to coat. Refrigerate 2 hours or up to 24 hours.

3 Spray grill pan with nonstick cooking spray; heat over medium-high heat. Remove pork from marinade; discard marinade. Cook pork 4 minutes per side or until just slightly pink in center. Place on plates; top with reserved 1 tablespoon marinade.

Nutrients Per Serving (½ of total recipe)

CALORIES 180   **TOTAL FAT** 5g   **CARBS** 4g   **NET CARBS** 3g
DIETARY FIBER 1g   **PROTEIN** 26g

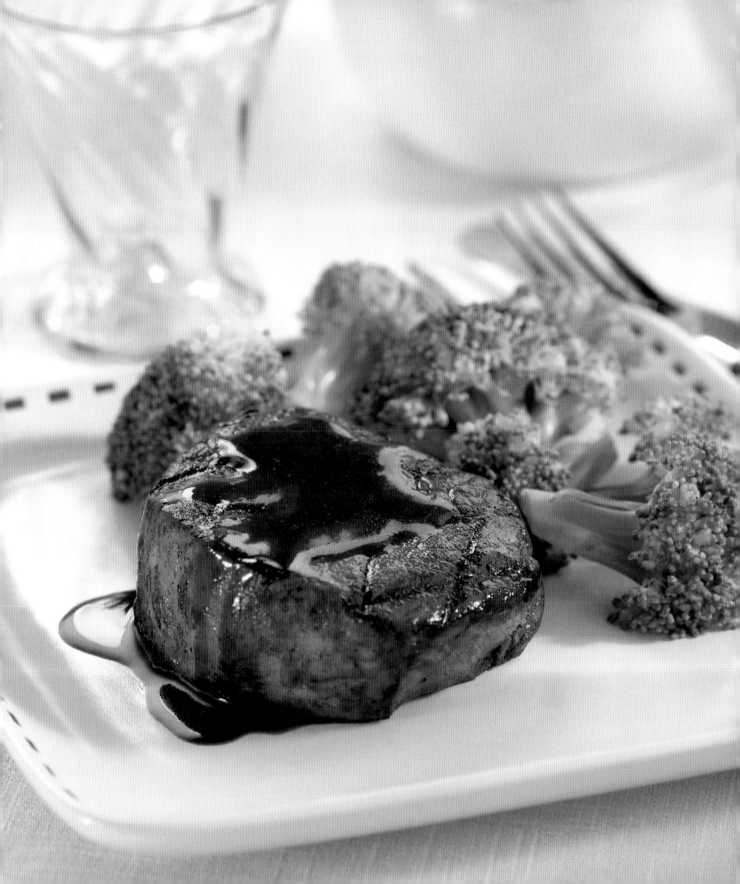

½ cup water

2 tablespoons Worcestershire sauce

2 tablespoons soy sauce

1 tablespoon chili powder

3 cloves garlic, minced, divided

2 teaspoons paprika

1½ teaspoons ground red pepper

1¼ teaspoons black pepper, divided

1 teaspoon onion powder

2 top sirloin steaks (about 8 ounces each, 1 inch thick)

3 tablespoons butter, divided

1 tablespoon olive oil

1 large onion, thinly sliced

8 ounces sliced mushrooms (white and shiitake or all white)

¼ teaspoon plus ⅛ teaspoon salt, divided

French Quarter Steaks
MAKES 2 SERVINGS

1 Combine water, Worcestershire sauce, soy sauce, chili powder, 2 cloves garlic, paprika, red pepper, 1 teaspoon black pepper and onion powder in small bowl; mix well. Place steaks in large resealable food storage bag; pour marinade over steaks. Seal bag; turn to coat. Marinate in refrigerator 1 to 3 hours.

2 Remove steaks from marinade 30 minutes before cooking; discard marinade and pat steaks dry with paper towel. Oil grid. Prepare grill for direct cooking.

3 While grill is preheating, heat 1 tablespoon butter and oil in large skillet over medium-high heat. Add onion; cook 5 minutes, stirring occasionally. Add mushrooms, ¼ teaspoon salt and remaining ¼ teaspoon black pepper; cook 10 minutes or until onion is golden brown and mushrooms are beginning to brown, stirring occasionally. Combine remaining 2 tablespoons butter, 1 clove garlic and ⅛ teaspoon salt in small skillet; cook over medium-low heat 3 minutes or until garlic begins to sizzle.

4 Grill steaks over medium-high heat 6 minutes; turn and grill 6 minutes for medium rare or until desired doneness. Brush both sides of steaks with garlic butter during last 2 minutes of cooking. Remove to plate and tent with foil; let rest 5 minutes. Serve steaks with onion and mushroom mixture.

Nutrients Per Serving (½ of total recipe)

CALORIES 520 **TOTAL FAT** 30g **CARBS** 9g **NET CARBS** 7g
DIETARY FIBER 2g **PROTEIN** 47g

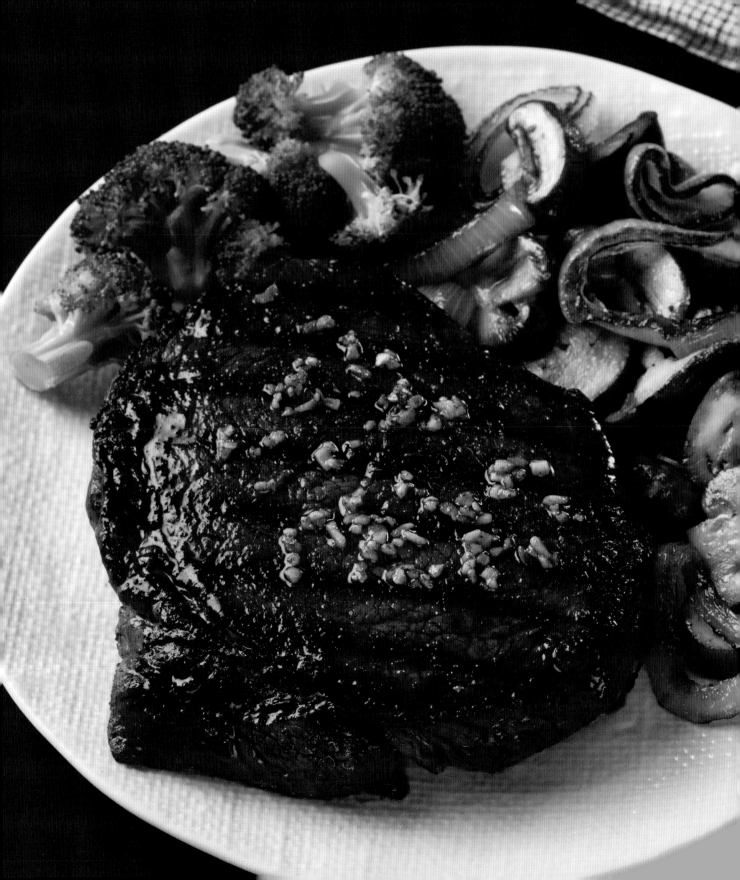

2 teaspoons whole black and pink peppercorns*

2 teaspoons coriander seeds

1 tablespoon peanut or canola oil

1 boneless beef top sirloin steak, about 1¼ inches thick (1¼ pounds)

2 teaspoons dark sesame oil

½ cup thinly sliced shallots or sweet onion

½ cup beef broth

2 tablespoons soy sauce

1 tablespoon dry sherry

2 tablespoons thinly sliced green onion or chopped fresh cilantro

You may use all black peppercorns if preferred.

Chinese Peppercorn Beef
MAKES 4 SERVINGS

1 Place peppercorns and coriander seeds in small resealable food storage bag; seal bag. Coarsely crush spices using meat mallet or bottom of heavy saucepan. Brush peanut oil over both sides of steak; sprinkle with peppercorn mixture, pressing lightly.

2 Heat large heavy skillet over medium-high heat. Add steak; cook 4 minutes without moving or until seared on bottom. Reduce heat to medium; turn steak and continue cooking 3 to 4 minutes for medium rare or until desired doneness. Transfer steak to cutting board; tent with foil and let stand while preparing sauce.

3 Add sesame oil to same skillet; heat over medium heat. Add shallots; cook and stir 3 minutes. Add broth, soy sauce and sherry; simmer about 5 minutes. Carve steak crosswise into thin slices. Spoon sauce over steak; sprinkle with green onion.

Nutrients Per Serving (¼ of total recipe)

CALORIES 330   TOTAL FAT 14g   CARBS 4g   NET CARBS 3g
DIETARY FIBER 1g   PROTEIN 43g

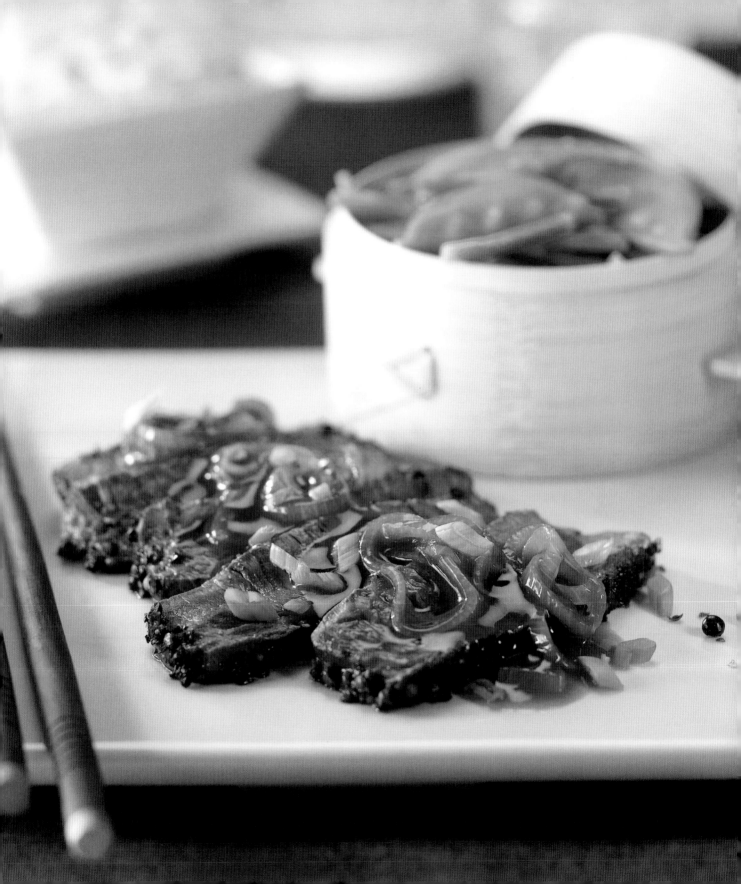

2 tablespoons olive oil

½ cup chopped green onions

12 ounces lean pork, cut into ¼-inch pieces

1 *each* red, yellow and green bell peppers, diced (about 2 cups)

1 teaspoon minced garlic

Salt and black pepper

1 cup sliced mushrooms

1 teaspoon ground cumin

1 teaspoon chili powder

½ teaspoon chipotle chile pepper (optional)

¼ cup (1 ounce) shredded Cheddar cheese

¼ cup sour cream

Pork and Peppers Mexican-Style
MAKES 4 SERVINGS

1 Heat oil in large skillet over medium-high heat. Add green onions; cook and stir 2 minutes. Add pork; cook and stir 5 minutes or until browned. Add bell peppers and garlic; cook and stir 5 minutes or until bell peppers begin to soften.

2 Season mixture in skillet with salt and black pepper. Add mushrooms, cumin, chili powder and chipotle pepper, if desired. Cook and stir 10 to 15 minutes until pork is cooked through and vegetables are tender. Serve with cheese and sour cream.

Nutrients Per Serving
(about 1¼ cups pork mixture, 1 tablespoon cheese and 1 tablespoon sour cream)

CALORIES 271 **TOTAL FAT** 16g **CARBS** 9g **NET CARBS** 6g
DIETARY FIBER 3g **PROTEIN** 22g

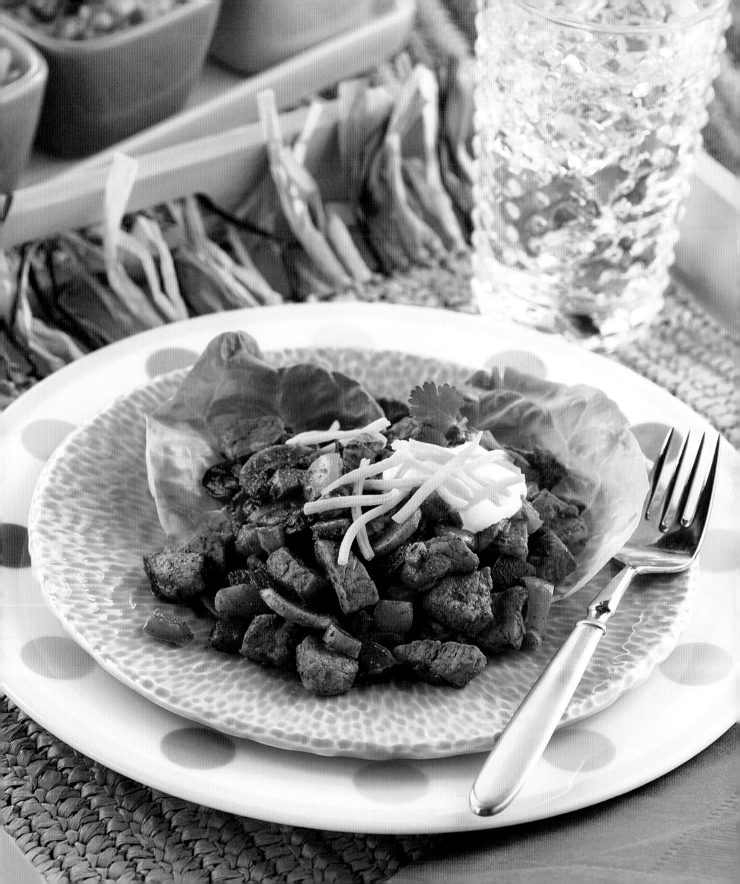

London Broil with Marinated Vegetables
MAKES 6 SERVINGS

¾ cup olive oil

¾ cup dry red wine

2 tablespoons finely chopped shallots

2 tablespoons red wine vinegar

2 teaspoons minced garlic

½ teaspoon dried thyme

½ teaspoon dried oregano

½ teaspoon dried basil

½ teaspoon black pepper

2 pounds top round London broil (1½ inches thick)

1 medium red onion, cut into ¼-inch-thick slices

1 package (8 ounces) sliced mushrooms

1 medium red bell pepper, cut into strips

1 medium zucchini, cut into ¼-inch-thick slices

1 Whisk oil, wine, shallots, vinegar, garlic, thyme, oregano, basil and black pepper in medium bowl until well blended. Combine London broil and ¾ cup marinade in large resealable food storage bag. Seal bag; turn to coat. Marinate in refrigerator at least 1 hour or up to 24 hours, turning bag once or twice.

2 Combine onion, mushrooms, bell pepper, zucchini and remaining marinade in separate large food storage bag. Seal bag and turn to coat. Refrigerate at least 1 hour or up to 24 hours, turning bag once or twice.

3 Preheat broiler. Remove beef from marinade and place on broiler pan; discard marinade. Broil 4 to 5 inches from heat about 9 minutes per side or until desired doneness. Let stand 10 minutes. Thinly slice beef.

4 Meanwhile, drain vegetables and arrange on broiler pan; discard marinade. Broil 4 to 5 inches from heat about 9 minutes or until edges of vegetables just begin to brown. Serve beef with vegetables.

Nutrients Per Serving (⅙ of total recipe)

CALORIES 385   **TOTAL FAT** 22g   **CARBS** 6g   **NET CARBS** 4g
DIETARY FIBER 2g   **PROTEIN** 37g

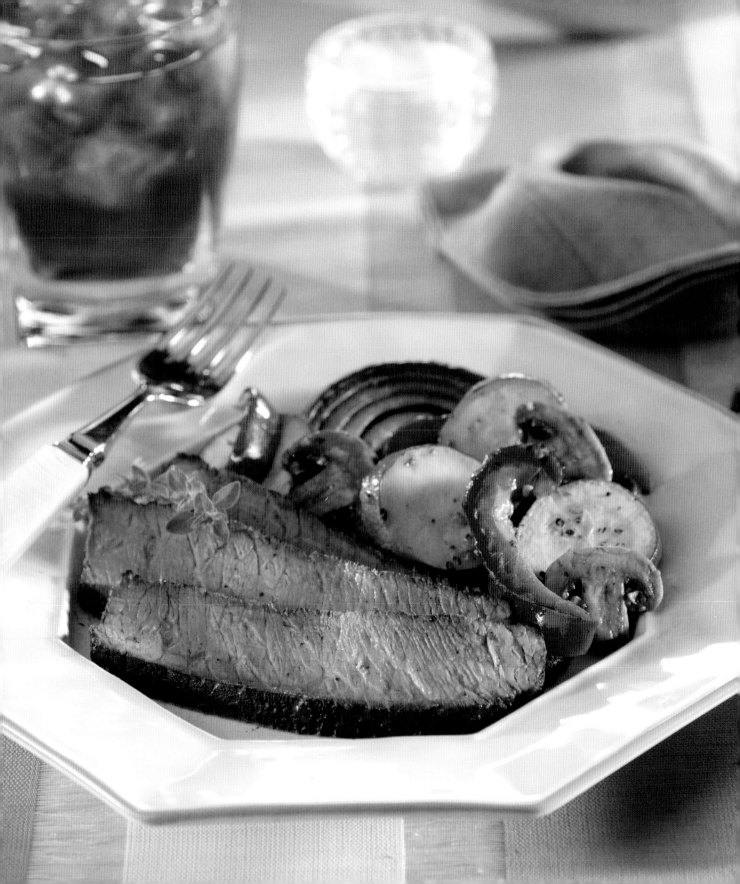

Pork

1½ teaspoons chili powder

½ teaspoon ground cumin

Salt and black pepper

1 pork tenderloin (about 1 pound)

1 teaspoon extra virgin olive oil

Salsa

2 medium tomatillos, husked* and diced

½ ripe medium avocado, diced

1 jalapeño pepper, seeded and finely chopped

1 clove garlic, minced

2 tablespoons finely chopped red onion

2 tablespoons chopped fresh cilantro

1 tablespoon lime juice

⅛ teaspoon salt

4 lime wedges (optional)

Remove the husk by pulling from the bottom to where it attaches at the stem. Wash before using.

Pork Tenderloin with Avocado-Tomatillo Salsa
MAKES 4 SERVINGS

1 Preheat oven to 425°F. Combine chili powder and cumin in small bowl. Sprinkle evenly all over pork and season with salt and black pepper; press to adhere spices.

2 Heat oil in large nonstick skillet over medium-high heat until hot. Add pork; cook 3 minutes. Turn and cook 2 to 3 minutes or until well browned. Place on foil-lined baking sheet; bake about 30 minutes or until barely pink in center (about 145°F). Let rest 5 minutes. Slice ¼ inch thick on the diagonal.

3 For salsa, combine tomatillos, avocado, jalapeño, garlic, onion, cilantro, lime juice and ⅛ teaspoon salt in medium bowl; toss gently to blend. Serve with pork and additional lime wedges, if desired.

Tip: Choose firm tomatillos with dry husks that are not too ragged. Store in a paper bag in refrigerator for up to 1 month.

Nutrients Per Serving (3 ounces pork and ¼ cup salsa)
CALORIES 174 **TOTAL FAT** 6g **CARBS** 4g **NET CARBS** 2g
DIETARY FIBER 2g **PROTEIN** 25g

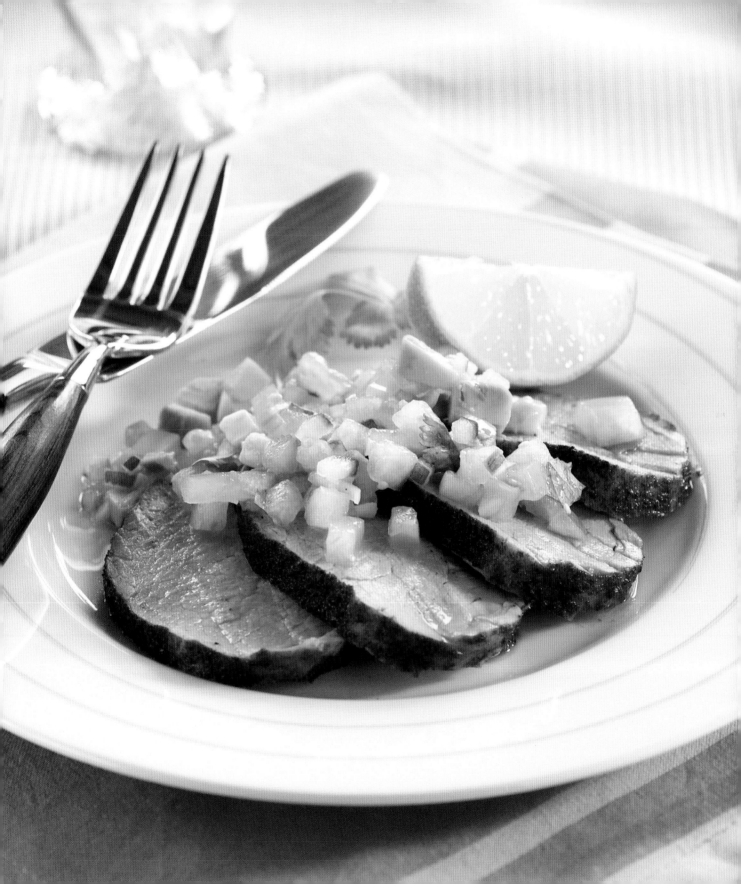

Flank Steak with Italian Salsa
MAKES 6 SERVINGS

2 tablespoons olive oil

2 teaspoons balsamic vinegar

1 lean flank steak (1½ pounds)

1 tablespoon minced garlic

¾ teaspoon salt, divided

¾ teaspoon black pepper, divided

1 cup diced plum tomatoes

⅓ cup chopped pitted kalamata olives

2 tablespoons chopped fresh basil

1 Whisk oil and vinegar in medium bowl until well blended. Place steak in shallow dish. Spread garlic over steak; sprinkle with ½ teaspoon salt and ½ teaspoon pepper. Spoon 2 tablespoons oil mixture over steak. Marinate in refrigerator at least 20 minutes or up to 2 hours.

2 Add tomatoes, olives, basil, remaining ¼ teaspoon salt and ¼ teaspoon pepper to remaining 2 teaspoons vinegar mixture in bowl; mix well.

3 Prepare grill for direct cooking or preheat broiler. Remove steak from marinade; discard marinade. (Leave garlic on steak.)

4 Grill steak over medium-high heat 5 to 6 minutes per side for medium rare. Remove to cutting board; tent with foil and let stand 5 minutes. Cut steak diagonally across the grain into thin slices. Serve with tomato mixture.

Nutrients Per Serving (⅙ of total recipe)
CALORIES 191 **TOTAL FAT** 11g **CARBS** 4g **NET CARBS** 3g
DIETARY FIBER 1g **PROTEIN** 18g

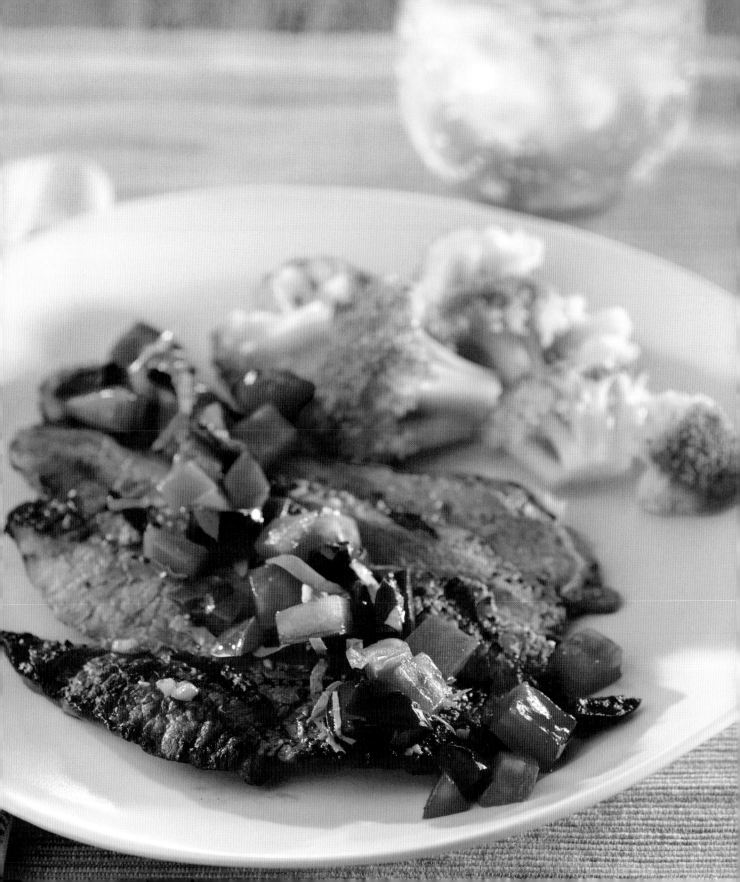

2 tablespoons Dijon
   mustard

1 teaspoon minced fresh
   tarragon

2 tablespoons lemon
   juice

⅓ cup chicken or
   vegetable broth

1½ to 2 pounds boneless
   pork loin

½ teaspoon freshly
   ground black
   pepper

1 teaspoon ground
   paprika

Pork Roast with
Dijon Tarragon Glaze
MAKES 4 TO 6 SERVINGS

Slow Cooker Directions

1 For glaze, combine mustard, tarragon, lemon juice
   and broth in small bowl; set aside. Sprinkle roast with
   pepper and paprika. Place roast in slow cooker. Spoon
   glaze evenly over roast.

2 Cover; cook on LOW 6 to 8 hours or on HIGH 3 to
   4 hours.

3 Remove roast from slow cooker; let stand 15 minutes
   before slicing.

Nutrients Per Serving
(3 ounces pork with 2 tablespoons glaze)

CALORIES 170   **TOTAL FAT** 6g   **CARBS** 2g   **NET CARBS** 1g
DIETARY FIBER 1g   **PROTEIN** 25g

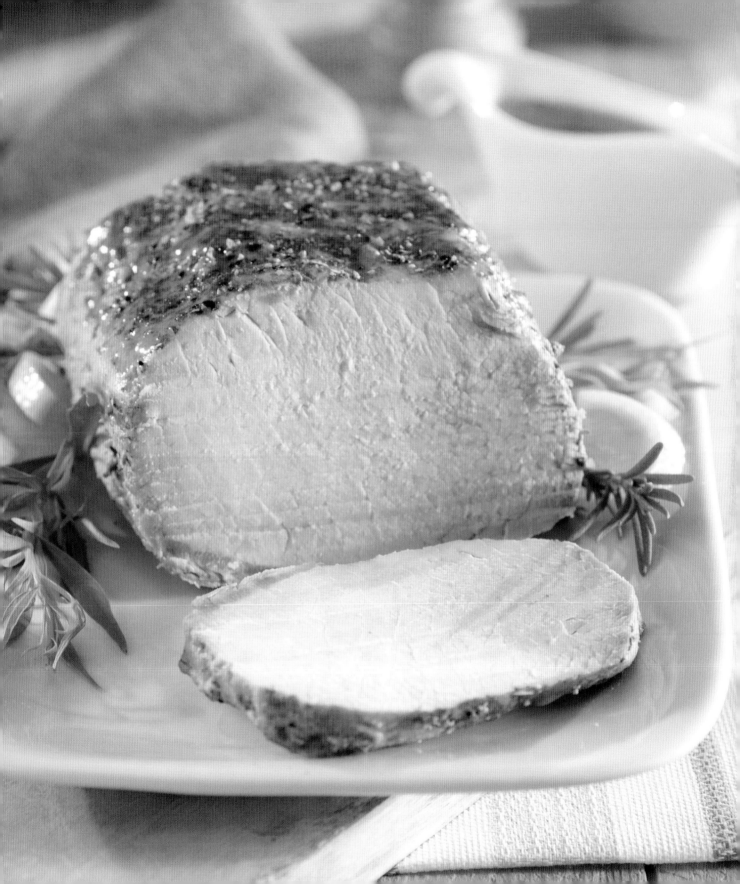

Brisket with Bacon, Blue Cheese and Onions

MAKES 10 SERVINGS

2 large sweet onions, sliced into ½-inch rounds

6 slices bacon, divided

1 flat-cut boneless beef brisket (about 3½ pounds)

Salt and black pepper

1 can (about 14 ounces) beef broth

1 teaspoon cracked black peppercorns

¾ cup crumbled blue cheese

Slow Cooker Directions

1 Coat 5- to 6-quart slow cooker with nonstick cooking spray. Line bottom with onion slices.

2 Heat large skillet over medium-high heat. Add bacon; cook until chewy, not crisp. Reserve drippings in skillet. Drain on paper towel-lined plate. Chop bacon.

3 Season brisket with salt and pepper. Sear brisket in bacon drippings on all sides. Remove to slow cooker.

4 Pour consommé into slow cooker. Sprinkle with peppercorns and half of bacon. Cover; cook on HIGH 5 to 7 hours.

5 Remove brisket to large cutting board; cover with foil. Let stand 10 to 15 minutes. Slice against the grain into ¾-inch slices.

6 Arrange brisket slices on plates; top with onions, blue cheese and remaining bacon. Season cooking liquid with salt and pepper; serve with brisket.

Nutrients Per Serving
(about 4 ounces brisket and ½ cup sauce)

CALORIES 470   **TOTAL FAT** 29g   **CARBS** 6g   **NET CARBS** 5g
DIETARY FIBER 1g   **PROTEIN** 45g

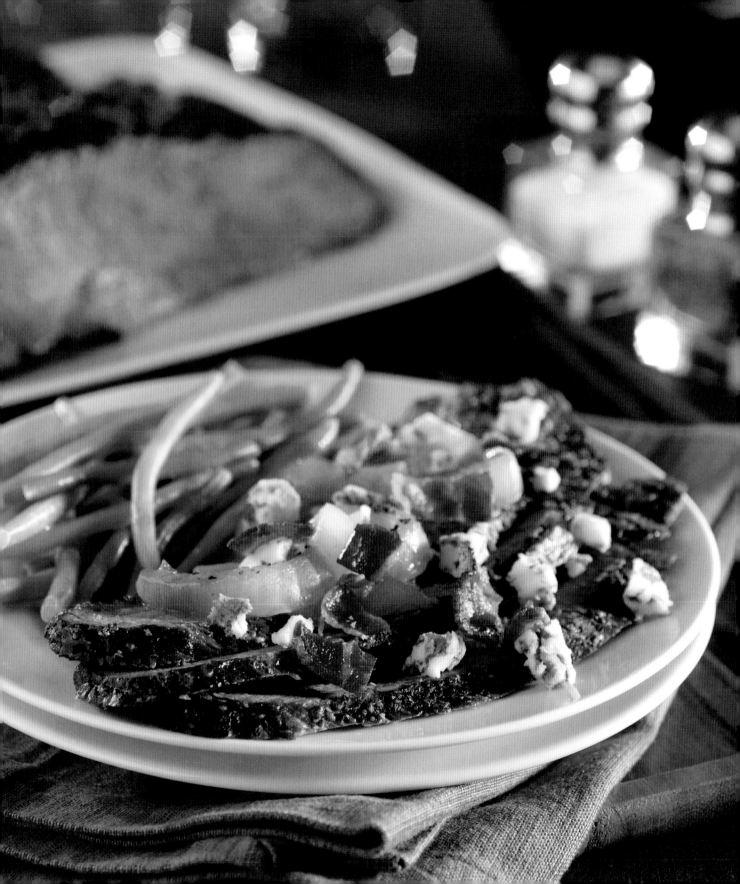

Pork with Cucumber Pico de Gallo

MAKES 4 SERVINGS

½ medium cucumber, seeded and finely chopped (4 ounces)

2 medium tomatillos, papery skin removed, rinsed and chopped

2 tablespoons chopped fresh cilantro leaves

⅛ teaspoon red pepper flakes

1 tablespoon lime juice

¼ teaspoon salt, divided

4 boneless center cut pork cutlets, trimmed of fat (about 1 pound)

¼ teaspoon coarsely ground black pepper

1 Combine cucumber, tomatillos, cilantro, red pepper flakes, lime juice and ⅛ teaspoon salt in medium bowl. Toss gently to blend; set aside.

2 Sprinkle pork chops evenly with black pepper and remaining ⅛ teaspoon salt.

3 Spray large nonstick skillet with nonstick cooking spray; heat over medium-high heat. Add pork; immediately reduce heat to medium. Cook 5 minutes. Turn and cook 4 to 5 minutes longer or until barely pink in center. Serve with cucumber mixture.

Note: To easily seed a cucumber, split cucumber in half lengthwise. Scoop out seeds with a teaspoon (this prevents the dish from being too watery and diluting the flavors).

Nutrients Per Serving
(3 ounces pork and ¼ cup cucumber mixture)

CALORIES 231 **TOTAL FAT** 13g **CARBS** 2g **NET CARBS** 1g
DIETARY FIBER 1g **PROTEIN** 23g

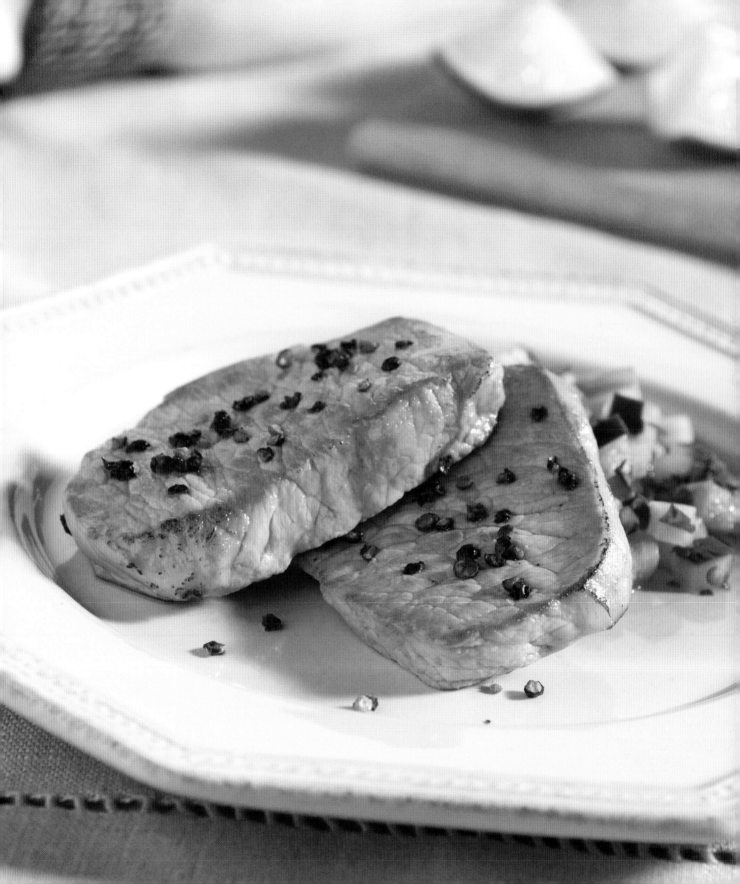

½ cup (1 stick) butter, softened

2 teaspoons chili powder

1 teaspoon minced garlic

1 teaspoon Dijon mustard

⅛ teaspoon ground red pepper or chipotle chile pepper

1 teaspoon black pepper

4 beef rib eye steaks

Salt

Rib Eye Steaks with Chile Butter

MAKES 4 SERVINGS

1 Beat butter, chili powder, garlic, mustard and red pepper in medium bowl until smooth. Place mixture on sheet of waxed paper. Roll mixture back and forth into 6-inch log using waxed paper. If butter is too soft, refrigerate up to 30 minutes. Wrap with waxed paper; refrigerate at least 1 hour or up to 2 days.

2 Oil grid. Prepare grill for direct cooking. Rub black pepper evenly over both sides of steaks; season with salt.

3 Place steaks on grid over medium-high heat. Grill, covered, 8 to 10 minutes or until desired doneness, turning occasionally. Slice chili butter; serve with steak.

Nutrients Per Serving (¼ of total recipe)

CALORIES 500   **TOTAL FAT** 37g   **CARBS** 2g   **NET CARBS** 1g
DIETARY FIBER 1g   **PROTEIN** 40g

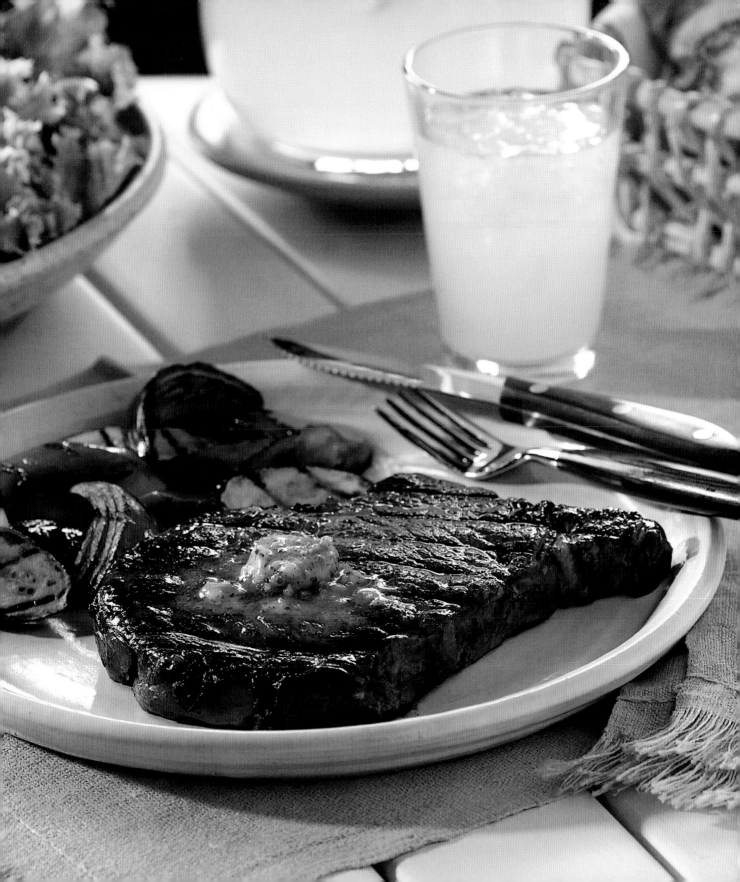

Korean Beef Short Ribs

MAKES 4 SERVINGS

2½ pounds beef chuck flanken-style short ribs, cut ⅜ to ½ inch thick*

¼ cup chopped green onions

¼ cup water

¼ cup soy sauce

2 teaspoons grated fresh ginger

2 teaspoons dark sesame oil

2 cloves garlic, minced

½ teaspoon black pepper

1 tablespoon sesame seeds, toasted

Flanken-style ribs can be ordered from your butcher. They are cross-cut short ribs sawed through the bones.

1 Place ribs in large resealable food storage bag. Combine green onions, water, soy sauce, ginger, oil, garlic and pepper in small bowl; pour over ribs. Seal bag; turn to coat. Marinate in refrigerator at least 4 hours or up to 8 hours, turning occasionally.

2 Prepare grill for direct cooking. Remove ribs from marinade; reserve marinade. Grill ribs, covered, over medium-high heat 5 minutes. Brush lightly with reserved marinade; turn and brush again. Discard remaining marinade. Continue to grill, covered, 5 to 6 minutes for medium (165°F) or to desired doneness. Sprinkle with sesame seeds.

Nutrients Per Serving (¼ of total recipe)

CALORIES 690 **TOTAL FAT** 60g **CARBS** 3g **NET CARBS** 2g
DIETARY FIBER 1g **PROTEIN** 31g

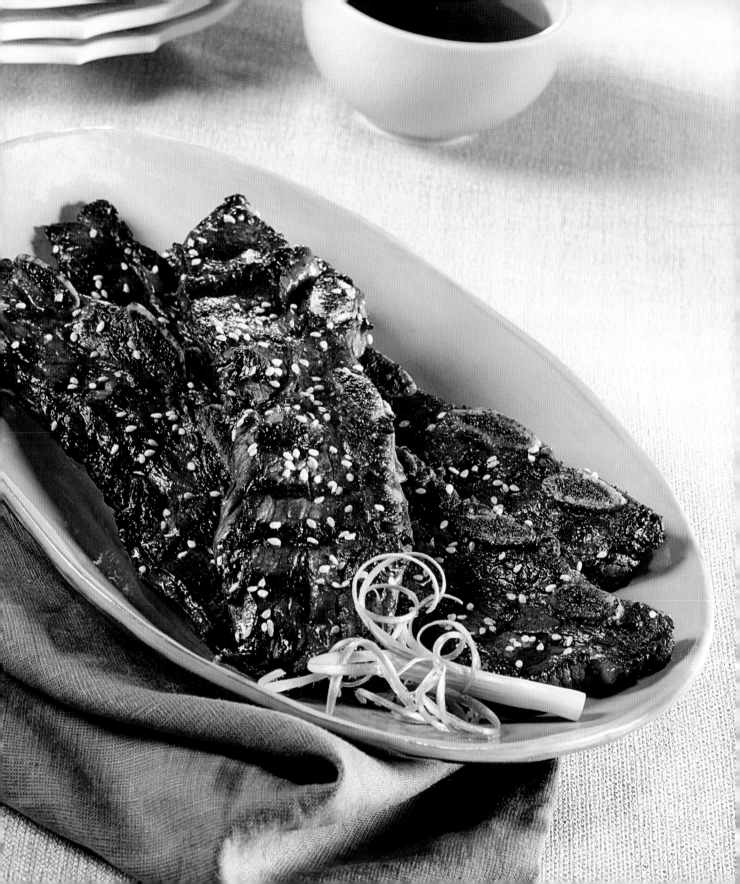

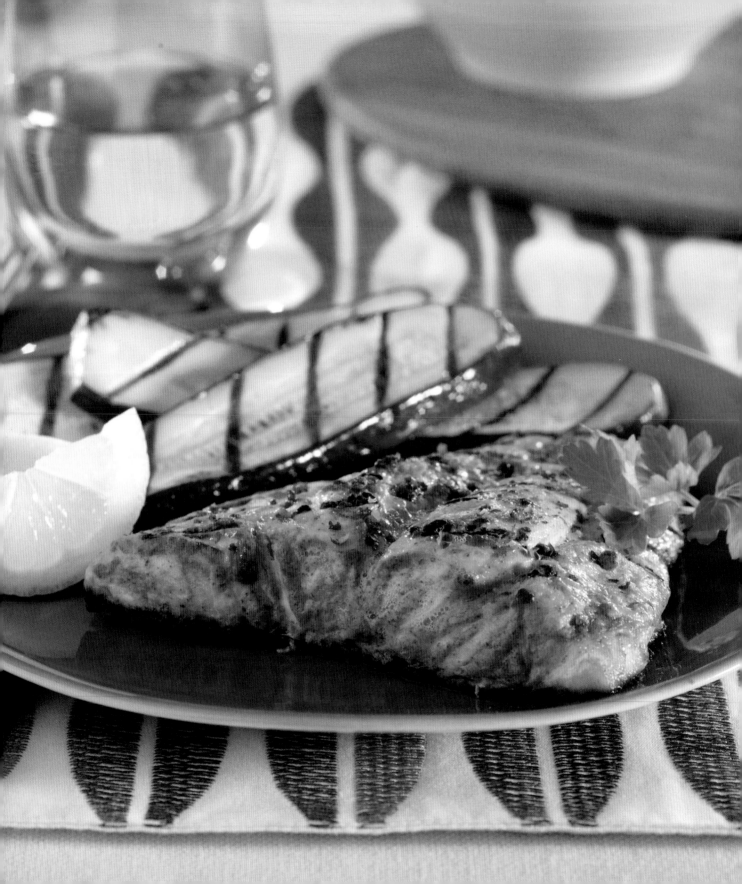

Fish and Seafood

Mustard-Grilled Red Snapper

MAKES 4 SERVINGS

1 Oil grid. Prepare grill for direct cooking.

2 Combine mustard, vinegar and red pepper in small bowl; mix well. Season fish with salt and black pepper; coat fish thoroughly with mustard mixture.

3 Grill fish, covered, over medium-high heat 8 minutes or until fish begins to flake easily when tested with fork, turning halfway through grilling time. Garnish with red peppercorns.

Nutrients Per Serving (1 fish fillet)

CALORIES 200 **TOTAL FAT** 3g **CARBS** 0g **NET CARBS** 0g
DIETARY FIBER 0g **PROTEIN** 35g

½ cup Dijon mustard

1 tablespoon red wine vinegar

1 teaspoon ground red pepper

4 red snapper fillets (about 6 ounces each)

Salt and black pepper

Red peppercorns (optional)

Spicy Butter

⅓ cup butter, melted

1 tablespoon finely chopped onion

2 to 3 teaspoons hot pepper sauce

1 teaspoon dried thyme

¼ teaspoon ground allspice

Scallion Butter

⅓ cup butter, melted

1 tablespoon finely chopped green onion top

1 tablespoon lemon juice

1 teaspoon freshly grated lemon peel

¼ teaspoon black pepper

Chili-Mustard Butter

⅓ cup butter, melted

1 tablespoon finely chopped onion

1 tablespoon Dijon mustard

1 teaspoon chili powder

Lobster

4 fresh or thawed frozen lobster tails (about 5 ounces each)

Lobster Tails with Tasty Butters
MAKES 4 SERVINGS

1 Prepare desired butter(s). Combine all ingredients for each butter in small bowl.

2 Oil grid. Prepare grill for direct cooking.

3 Rinse lobster tails in cold water. Butterfly tails by cutting lengthwise through centers of hard top shells and meat. Cut to, but not through, bottoms of shells. Press shell halves of tails apart with fingers. Brush lobster meat with butter mixture.

4 Place tails on grid, meat side down. Grill, uncovered, over medium-high heat 4 minutes. Turn tails meat side up. Brush with butter mixture; grill 4 to 5 minutes or until lobster meat turns opaque.

5 Heat remaining butter mixture, stirring occasionally. Serve with lobster for dipping.

Nutrients Per Serving
(1 lobster tail and about 2 tablespoons butter)
CALORIES 278   TOTAL FAT 18g   CARBS 1g   NET CARBS 0g
DIETARY FIBER 1g   PROTEIN 27g

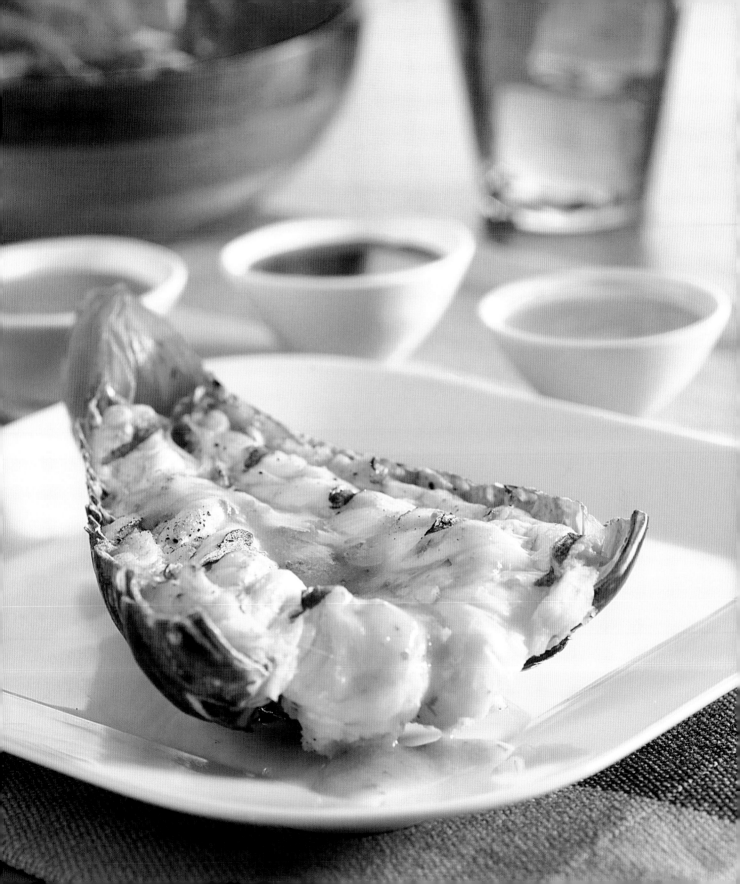

Pan-Seared Halibut Steaks with Avocado Salsa

MAKES 4 SERVINGS

4 tablespoons chipotle salsa, divided

½ teaspoon salt, divided

4 small (4 to 5 ounces each) *or* 2 large (8 to 10 ounces each) halibut steaks, cut ¾ inch thick

½ cup diced tomato

½ ripe avocado, diced

2 tablespoons chopped fresh cilantro (optional)

Lime wedges (optional)

1 Combine 2 tablespoons salsa and ¼ teaspoon salt in small bowl; spread over both sides of halibut.

2 Heat large nonstick skillet over medium heat. Add halibut; cook 4 to 5 minutes per side or until fish is opaque in center.

3 Meanwhile, combine remaining 2 tablespoons salsa, ¼ teaspoon salt, tomato, avocado and cilantro, if desired, in small bowl; mix well. Spoon over cooked fish. Garnish with lime wedges.

Nutrients Per Serving
(1 halibut steak and 3 tablespoons salsa)

CALORIES 150 **TOTAL FAT** 5g **CARBS** 4g **NET CARBS** 2g
DIETARY FIBER 2g **PROTEIN** 22g

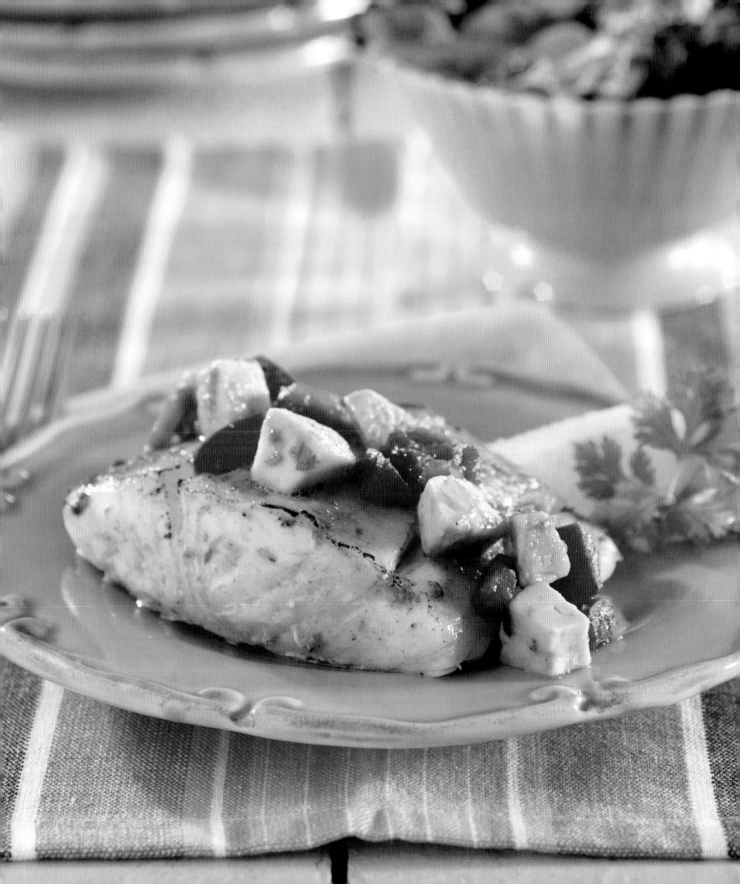

¼ cup reduced-sodium
   soy sauce

2 tablespoons lime juice

1 tablespoon dark
   sesame oil

1 teaspoon grated fresh
   ginger

⅛ teaspoon red pepper
   flakes

32 medium raw shrimp
   (about 8 ounces
   total), peeled,
   deveined, rinsed
   and patted dry

2 medium zucchini, cut
   in half lengthwise
   and thinly sliced

6 green onions,
   trimmed and halved
   lengthwise

12 grape tomatoes

Shrimp and Veggie Skillet Toss
MAKES 4 SERVINGS

1 Whisk soy sauce, lime juice, oil, ginger and red pepper
   flakes in small bowl; set aside.

2 Spray large nonstick skillet with nonstick cooking spray;
   heat over medium-high heat. Add shrimp; cook and
   stir 3 minutes or until shrimp are opaque. Remove from
   skillet.

3 Spray same skillet with cooking spray. Add zucchini;
   cook and stir 4 to 6 minutes or just until crisp-tender.
   Add green onions and tomatoes; cook 1 to 2 minutes.
   Add shrimp, cook 1 minute. Transfer to large bowl.

4 Add soy sauce mixture to skillet; bring to a boil. Remove
   from heat. Stir in shrimp and vegetables; gently toss.

Nutrients Per Serving
(1 cup shrimp mixture and 1 tablespoon sauce)
CALORIES 110   **TOTAL FAT** 5g   **CARBS** 10g   **NET CARBS** 8g
DIETARY FIBER 2g   **PROTEIN** 11g

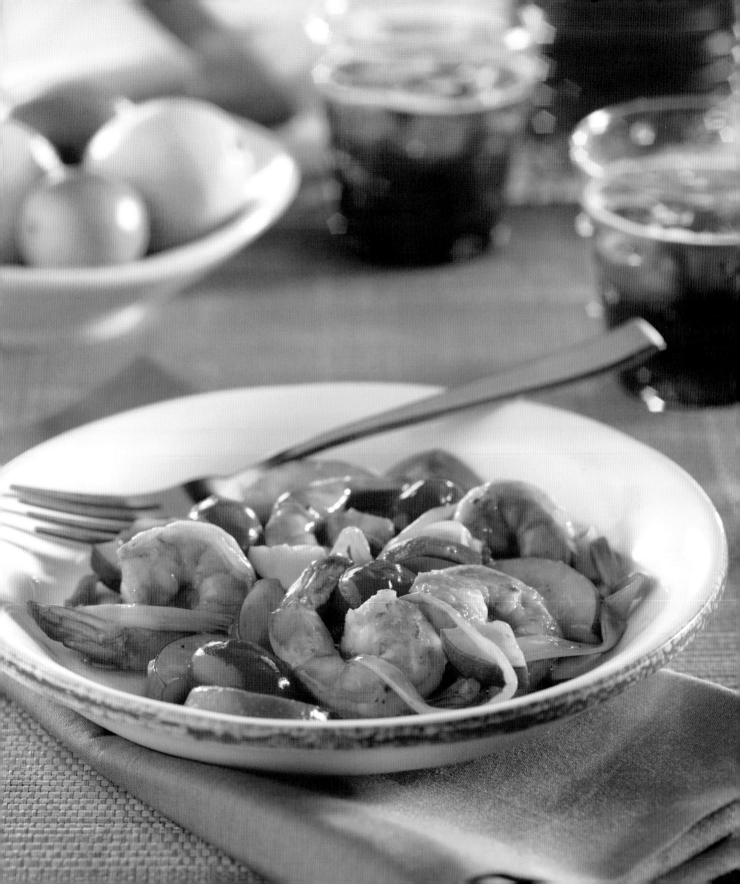

Hazelnut-Coated Salmon Steaks
MAKES 4 SERVINGS

¼ cup hazelnuts

4 salmon steaks (about 5 ounces each)

1 tablespoon olive oil

1 tablespoon Dijon mustard

½ teaspoon salt

¼ teaspoon dried thyme

⅛ teaspoon black pepper

1 Preheat oven to 375°F. Spread hazelnuts on ungreased baking sheet; bake 8 minutes or until lightly browned. Immediately transfer nuts to clean, dry dish towel. Fold towel over nuts; rub vigorously to remove as much of skins as possible. Finely chop hazelnuts in food processor or with knife.

2 *Increase oven temperature to 450°F.* Place salmon in single layer in baking dish. Combine oil, mustard, salt, thyme and pepper in small bowl; brush over salmon. Top with hazelnuts, pressing to adhere.

3 Bake 14 to 16 minutes or until salmon begins to flake when tested with fork.

Nutrients Per Serving (1 salmon steak)

CALORIES 350 **TOTAL FAT** 23g **CARBS** 2g **NET CARBS** 1g
DIETARY FIBER 1g **PROTEIN** 30g

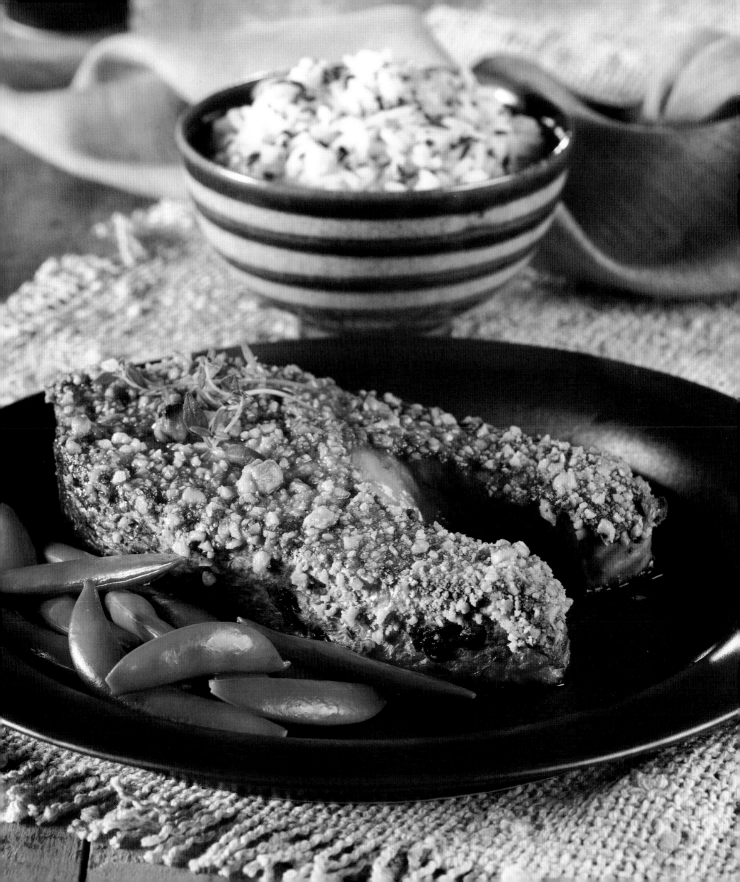

4 whole trout (each about 8 ounces), cleaned

¼ cup olive oil

¼ cup dry white wine

2 tablespoons minced frsh chives

2 tablespoons chopped fresh parsley

½ teaspoon salt

⅛ teaspoon black pepper

¼ cup (½ stick) butter, softened

¼ cup pine nuts, finely chopped

1 lemon, cut into wedges (optional)

Broiled Trout with Pine Nut Butter

MAKES 4 SERVINGS

1 Place trout in large resealable food storage bag. Whisk oil, wine, chives, parsley, salt and pepper in small bowl. Pour over fish; seal bag. Marinate 30 minutes or refrigerate up to 2 hours, turning bag occasionally to distribute marinade.

2 Combine butter and pine nuts in small bowl; stir until well blended. Cover; let stand at room temperature until ready to use.

3 Preheat broiler; spray broiler pan with nonstick cooking spray. Remove fish from marinade; reserve marinade. Place fish on prepared pan.

4 Broil 4 to 6 inches from heat 4 minutes; turn fish over. Brush with marinade; continue broiling 4 to 6 minutes or until fish turns opaque and just begins to flake with tested with fork. Transfer fish to serving platter. Serve with butter mixture and lemon wedges.

Nutrients Per Serving (¼ of total recipe)

CALORIES 540   **TOTAL FAT** 42g   **CARBS** 1g   **NET CARBS** 1g
DIETARY FIBER 0g   **PROTEIN** 26g

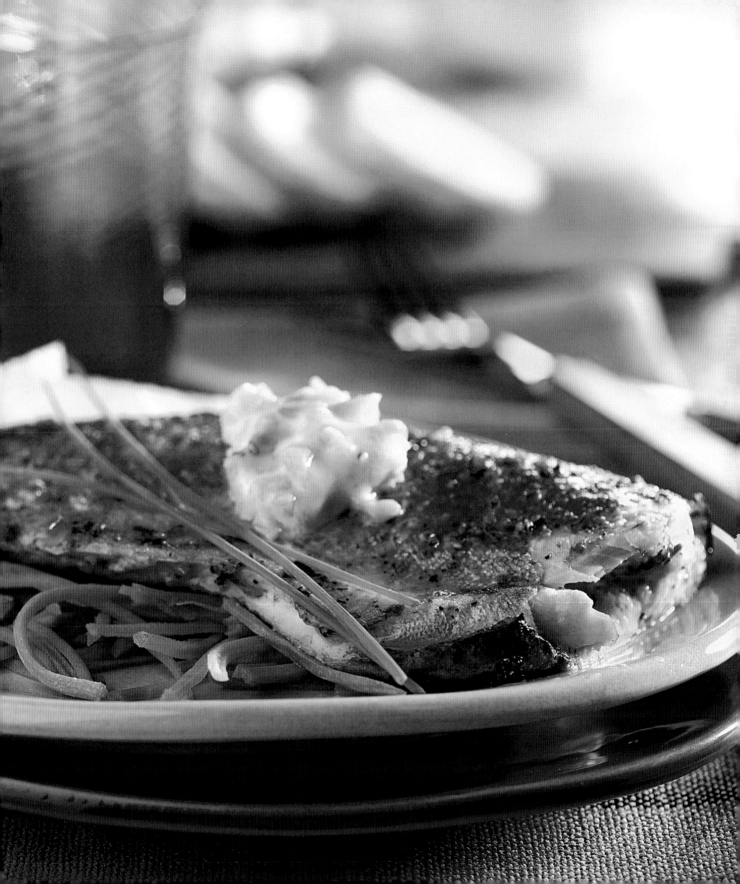

Seared Scallops over Garlic-Lemon Spinach

MAKES 4 SERVINGS

1 tablespoon olive oil

1 pound sea scallops (approximately 12), patted dry*

¼ teaspoon salt

⅛ teaspoon black pepper

2 cloves garlic, minced

1 shallot, minced

1 package (6 ounces) baby spinach

1 tablespoon fresh lemon juice

Lemon wedges (optional)

Make sure scallops are dry before putting them in the pan so they can get a golden crust.

1 Heat oil in large nonstick skillet over medium-high heat. Add scallops; sprinkle with salt and pepper. Cook 2 to 3 minutes per side or until golden. Remove to large plate; keep warm.

2 Add garlic and shallot to skillet; cook and stir 45 seconds or just until fragrant. Add spinach; cook 2 minutes or until spinach just begins to wilt, stirring occasionally. Remove from heat; stir in lemon juice.

3 Serve scallops over spinach. Garnish with lemon wedges.

Nutrients Per Serving (3 scallops and ¼ cup spinach)

CALORIES 172 **TOTAL FAT** 5g **CARBS** 3g **NET CARBS** 2g
DIETARY FIBER 1g **PROTEIN** 28g

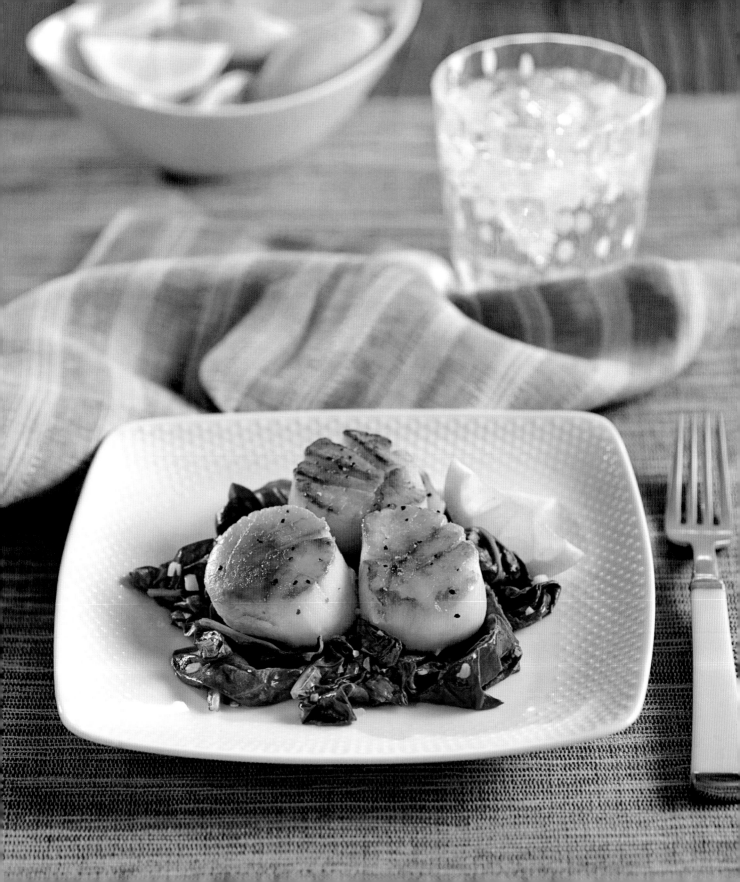

¼ cup soy sauce

2 tablespoons lime juice

1 tablespoon grated
   fresh ginger

1 tablespoon minced
   garlic

¼ teaspoon black
   pepper

4 salmon fillets
   (5 to 6 ounces each)

2 tablespoons minced
   green onion

Soy-Marinated Salmon
MAKES 4 SERVINGS

1 Combine soy sauce, lime juice, ginger, garlic and pepper in medium bowl; mix well. Reserve ¼ cup mixture for serving; set aside. Place salmon in large resealable food storage bag. Pour remaining mixture over salmon; seal bag and turn to coat. Marinate in refrigerator 2 to 4 hours, turning occasionally.

2 Prepare grill or preheat broiler. Remove salmon from marinade; discard marinade.

3 Grill or broil salmon 10 minutes or until fish begins to flake when tested with fork. (To broil, place salmon on foil-lined baking sheet sprayed with nonstick cooking spray.) Brush with some of reserved marinade mixture; sprinkle with green onion.

Nutrients Per Serving (1 salmon fillet)

CALORIES 310   **TOTAL FAT** 19g   **CARBS** 2g   **NET CARBS** 2g
DIETARY FIBER 0g   **PROTEIN** 31g

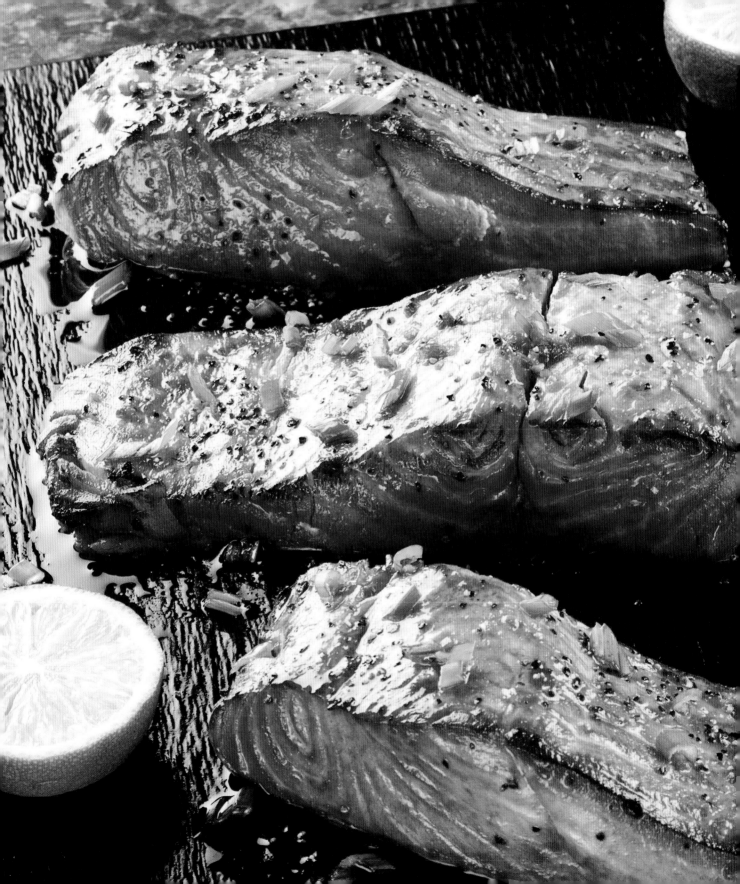

Tarragon Aioli Sauce

- ⅓ cup sour cream
- 1½ tablespoons mayonnaise
- 1 tablespoon milk
- ½ teaspoon dried tarragon
- ¼ teaspoon salt
- ⅛ teaspoon black pepper

Burgers

- 1 can (6 ounces) pink salmon, drained
- ¼ cup almond flour
- ⅓ cup chopped green onions
- ¼ cup chopped fresh cilantro
- 2 egg whites
- 2 tablespoons lime juice
- ¼ teaspoon salt
- ⅛ teaspoon ground red pepper

Salmon Burgers with Tarragon Aioli Sauce

MAKES 4 SERVINGS

1 For sauce, combine sour cream, mayonnaise, milk, tarragon, ¼ teaspoon salt and black pepper in medium bowl; stir to blend. Refrigerate until ready to use.

2 For burgers, combine salmon, almond flour, green onions, cilantro, egg whites, lime juice, ¼ teaspoon salt and red pepper in large bowl; mix well.

3 Spray large nonstick skillet with nonstick cooking spray; heat over medium heat. Spoon equal amounts of salmon mixture into four mounds in skillet. Using a flat spatula, flatten each mound. Cook 3 minutes per side or until golden. Serve with sauce.

Nutrients Per Serving
(1 burger and 2 tablespoons sauce)

CALORIES 190 **TOTAL FAT** 14g **CARBS** 6g **NET CARBS** 4g
DIETARY FIBER 2g **PROTEIN** 11g

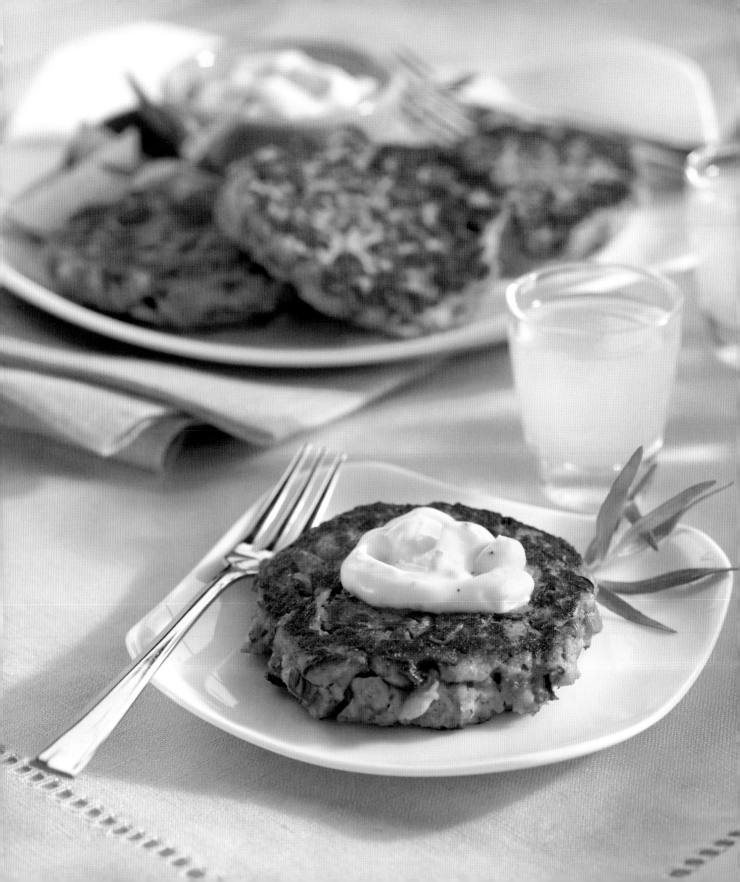

Grilled Scallops and Vegetables with Cilantro Sauce
MAKES 4 SERVINGS

1 teaspoon hot chili oil

1 teaspoon dark sesame oil

1 green onion, chopped

1 tablespoon finely chopped fresh ginger

1 cup chicken broth

1 cup chopped fresh cilantro

1 pound raw or thawed frozen sea scallops

2 medium zucchini, cut into ½-inch slices

2 medium yellow squash, cut into ½-inch slices

1 medium yellow onion, cut into wedges

8 large mushrooms

1 If using wooden skewers, soak in water 25 to 30 minutes before using to prevent burning. Spray grid with nonstick cooking spray. Prepare grill for direct cooking.

2 Heat chili oil and sesame oil in small saucepan over medium-low heat. Add green onion; cook and stir about 15 seconds or just until fragrant. Add ginger; cook and stir 1 minute. Stir in broth; bring to a boil. Cook until liquid is reduced by half; cool slightly. Pour into blender or food processor; add cilantro and blend until smooth. (Or add cilantro to saucepan and use hand-held immersion blender to blend mixture until smooth.)

3 Thread scallops and vegetables onto four 12-inch skewers.

4 Grill over medium-high heat about 8 minutes per side or until scallops turn opaque. Serve hot with cilantro sauce.

Nutrients Per Serving (1 skewer and ¼ of sauce)

CALORIES 194   TOTAL FAT 7g   CARBS 11g   NET CARBS 8g
DIETARY FIBER 3g   PROTEIN 23g

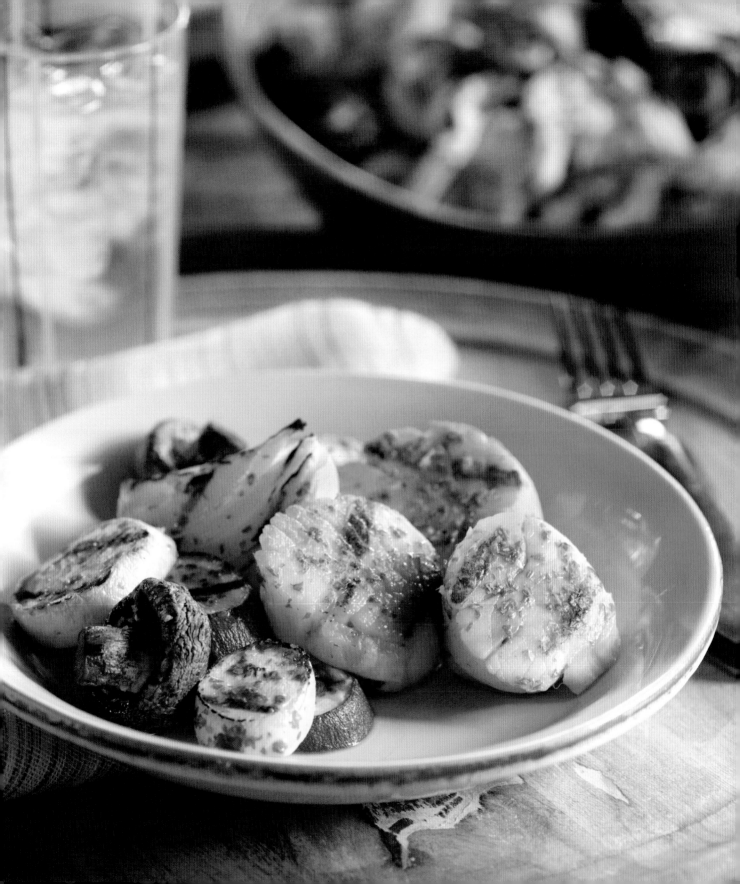

Szechuan Tuna Steaks

MAKES 4 SERVINGS

4 tuna steaks (6 ounces each), 1 inch thick

¼ cup dry sherry or sake

¼ cup soy sauce

1 tablespoon dark sesame oil

1 teaspoon hot chili oil *or* ¼ teaspoon red pepper flakes

1 clove garlic, minced

3 tablespoons chopped fresh cilantro (optional)

1 Place tuna in single layer in large shallow glass dish. Combine sherry, soy sauce, sesame oil, hot chili oil and garlic in small bowl. Reserve ¼ cup soy sauce mixture at room temperature. Pour remaining soy sauce mixture over fish; cover and marinate in refrigerator 40 minutes, turning once.

2 Spray grid with nonstick cooking spray. Prepare grill for direct cooking. Drain fish, discarding marinade.

3 Grill fish, uncovered, over medium-high heat 6 minutes or until tuna is seared but still feels somewhat soft in center,* turning halfway through grilling time. Remove to cutting board. Cut into thin slices; drizzle with reserved soy sauce mixture. Garnish with cilantro.

Tuna becomes dry and tough if overcooked. Cook to medium doneness for best results.

Nutrients Per Serving
(1 tuna steak and 1 tablespoon sauce)

CALORIES 284   TOTAL FAT 11g   CARBS 2g   NET CARBS 1g
DIETARY FIBER 1g   PROTEIN 40g

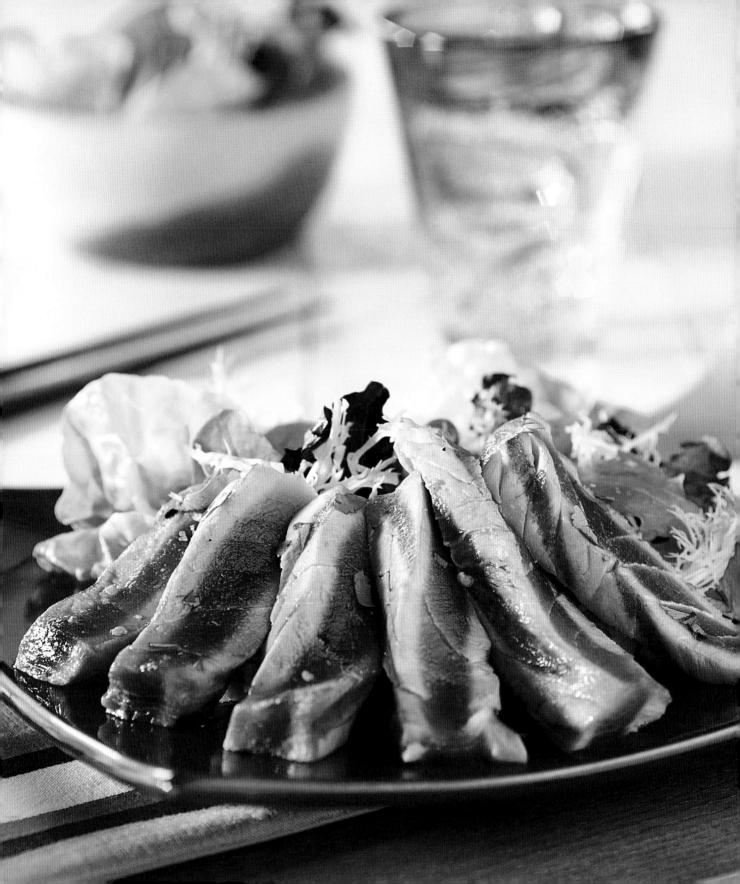

1 can (about 6 ounces) lump white crabmeat, drained

6 eggs

¼ teaspoon salt

¼ teaspoon black pepper

¼ teaspoon hot pepper sauce

1 tablespoon olive oil

1 green bell pepper, finely chopped

2 cloves garlic, minced

1 plum tomato, seeded and finely chopped

Spicy Crabmeat Frittata

MAKES 4 SERVINGS

1 Preheat broiler. Pick out and discard any shell or cartilage from crabmeat; break up large pieces of crabmeat.

2 Beat eggs in medium bowl. Add crabmeat, salt, black pepper and hot pepper sauce; mix well.

3 Heat oil in large ovenproof skillet over medium-high heat. Add bell pepper and garlic; cook and stir 3 minutes or until tender. Add tomato; cook and stir 1 minute. Stir in egg mixture; cook over medium-low heat 7 minutes or until eggs begin to set around edges.

4 Transfer skillet to broiler. Broil 4 inches from heat source 1 to 2 minutes or until frittata is golden brown and center is set.

Nutrients Per Serving (¼ of frittata)

CALORIES 187   **TOTAL FAT** 11g   **CARBS** 4g   **NET CARBS** 3g   **DIETARY FIBER** 1g   **PROTEIN** 17g

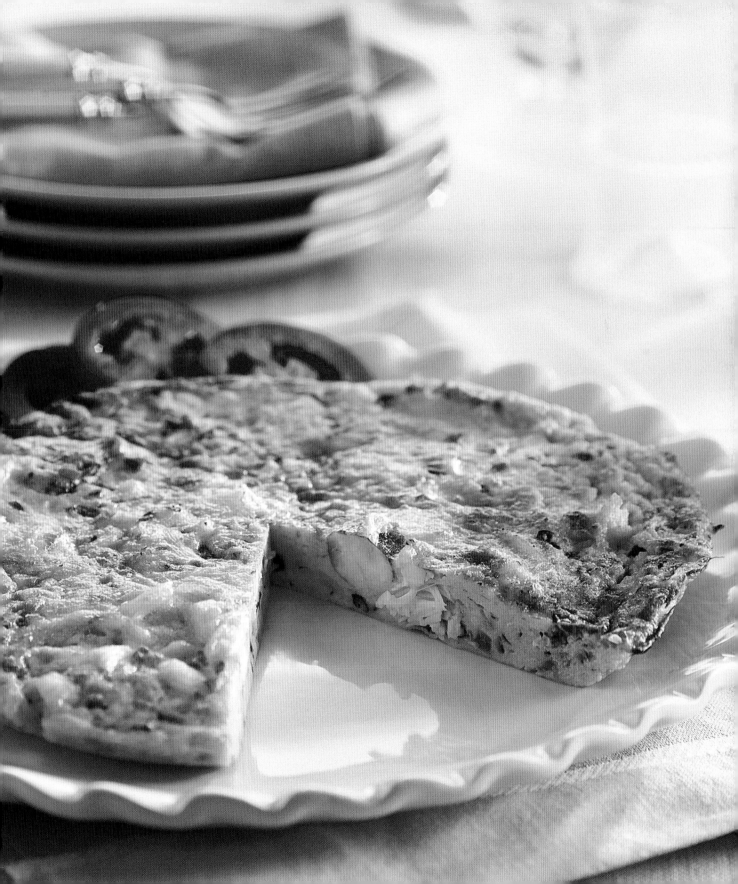

1 pound bok choy or
   napa cabbage,
   chopped
1 cup broccoli slaw mix
2 salmon fillets
   (4 to 6 ounces
   each)
½ teaspoon black
   pepper
¼ teaspoon salt
2 tablespoons olive oil,
   divided
1 teaspoon sesame
   seeds

Pan-Cooked Bok Choy Salmon
MAKES 2 SERVINGS

1 Combine bok choy and broccoli slaw mix in colander; rinse and drain well.

2 Sprinkle salmon with pepper and salt. Heat 1 tablespoon oil in large skillet over medium heat. Add salmon; cook 3 minutes per side. Remove salmon from skillet.

3 Add remaining 1 tablespoon oil and sesame seeds to skillet; stir to toast sesame seeds. Add bok choy mixture; cook and stir 3 to 4 minutes.

4 Return salmon to skillet. Reduce heat to low; cover and cook 4 minutes or until salmon begins to flake when tested with fork. Season with additional salt and pepper, if desired.

Nutrients Per Serving (½ of recipe)

CALORIES 410   **TOTAL FAT** 30g   **CARBS** 8g   **NET CARBS** 5g
DIETARY FIBER 3g   **PROTEIN** 28g

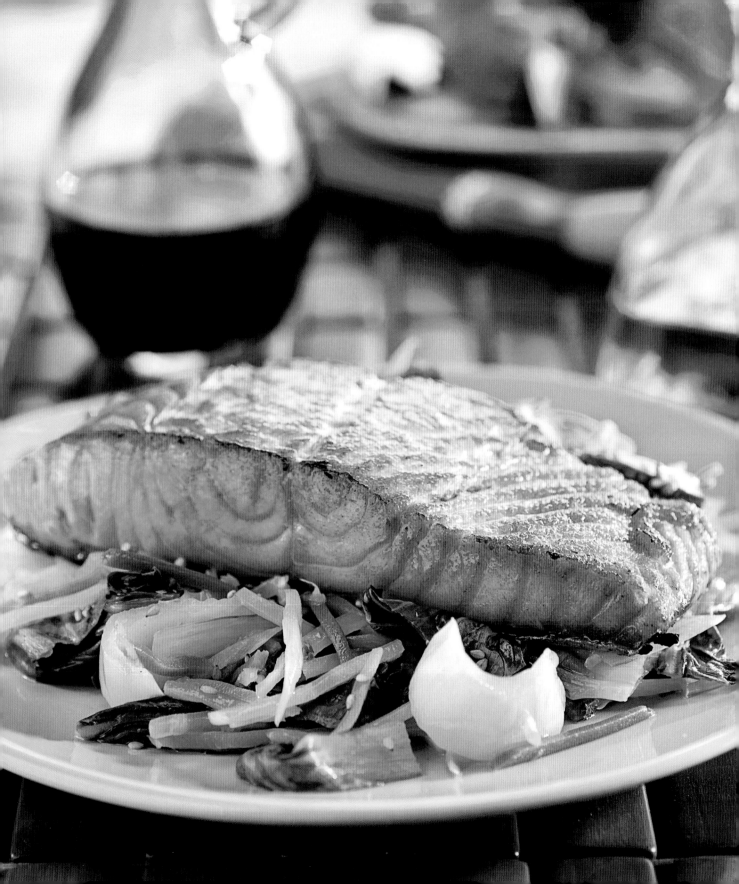

Tilapia with Spinach and Feta

MAKES 2 SERVINGS

1 teaspoon olive oil

1 clove garlic, minced

4 cups baby spinach

¼ teaspoon salt

2 skinless tilapia fillets or other mild white fish (4 ounces each)

¼ teaspoon black pepper

2 ounces feta cheese, cut into 2 (3-inch) pieces

1 Preheat oven to 350°F. Spray baking sheet with nonstick cooking spray.

2 Heat oil in medium skillet over medium-low heat. Add garlic; cook and stir 30 seconds. Add spinach; cook just until wilted, stirring occasionally. Stir in salt.

3 Arrange tilapia on prepared baking sheet; sprinkle with pepper. Place 1 piece of cheese on each fillet; top with spinach mixture. Fold one end of each fillet up and over filling; secure with toothpick. Repeat with opposite end of each fillet.

4 Bake 20 minutes or until fish begins to flake when tested with fork.

Nutrients Per Serving (½ of total recipe)

CALORIES 193 **TOTAL FAT** 9g **CARBS** 3g **NET CARBS** 2g
DIETARY FIBER 1g **PROTEIN** 26g

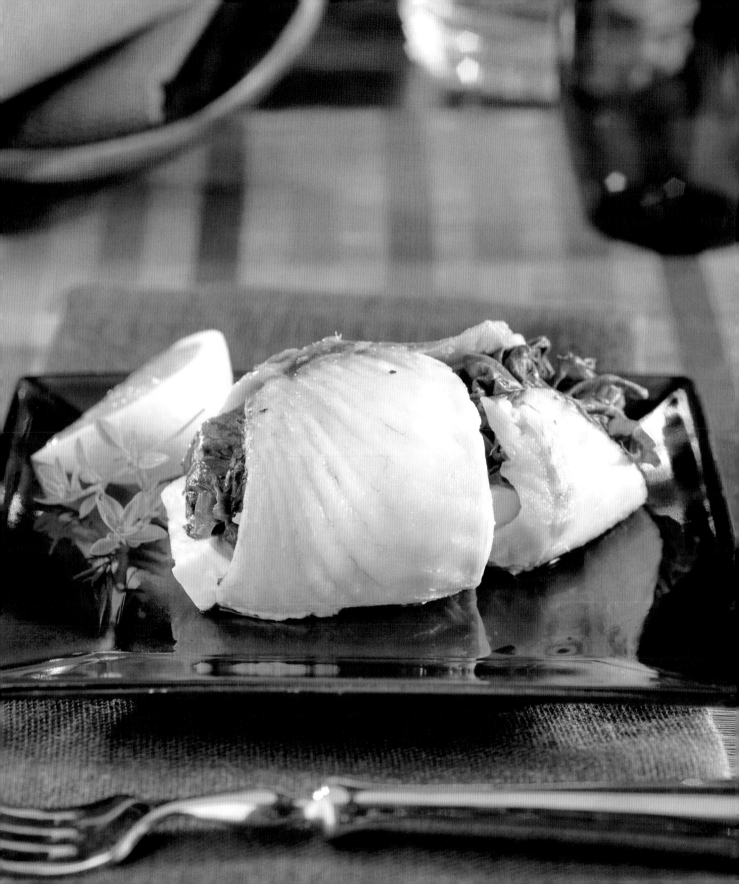

Miso Salmon over Garlicky Spinach
MAKES 4 SERVINGS

1½ tablespoons red miso

1 teaspoon minced ginger

¼ teaspoon salt

¼ teaspoon red pepper flakes

1 tablespoon plus 2 teaspoons water, divided

4 skinless salmon fillets (5 ounces each)

4 cloves garlic, minced

1 bag (10 ounces) fresh spinach leaves or baby spinach

1 Preheat broiler. Combine miso, ginger, salt and red pepper flakes in medium bowl; stir in 2 teaspoons water until blended. Reserve ½ teaspoon mixture in small bowl; spread remaining mixture over tops of salmon fillets. Place salmon on broiler pan or baking sheet.

2 Broil 4 to 5 inches from heat source 5 to 6 minutes or until salmon is opaque in center.

3 Meanwhile, spray large skillet with nonstick cooking spray; heat over medium heat. Add garlic; cook and stir 2 minutes. Stir remaining 1 tablespoon water into reserved miso mixture; mix well. Stir into garlic in skillet. Add spinach to skillet; cook 1 to 2 minutes or just until wilted, turning with tongs constantly. Transfer to serving plates; top with salmon.

Nutrients Per Serving (¼ of total recipe)
CALORIES 330 **TOTAL FAT** 19g **CARBS** 5g **NET CARBS** 3g
DIETARY FIBER 2g **PROTEIN** 32g

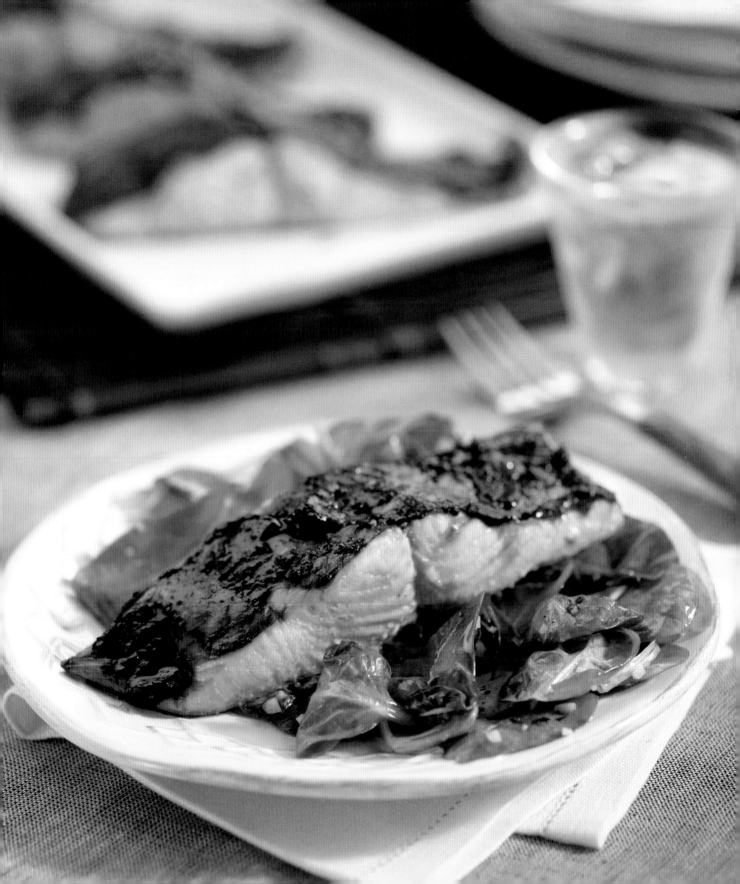

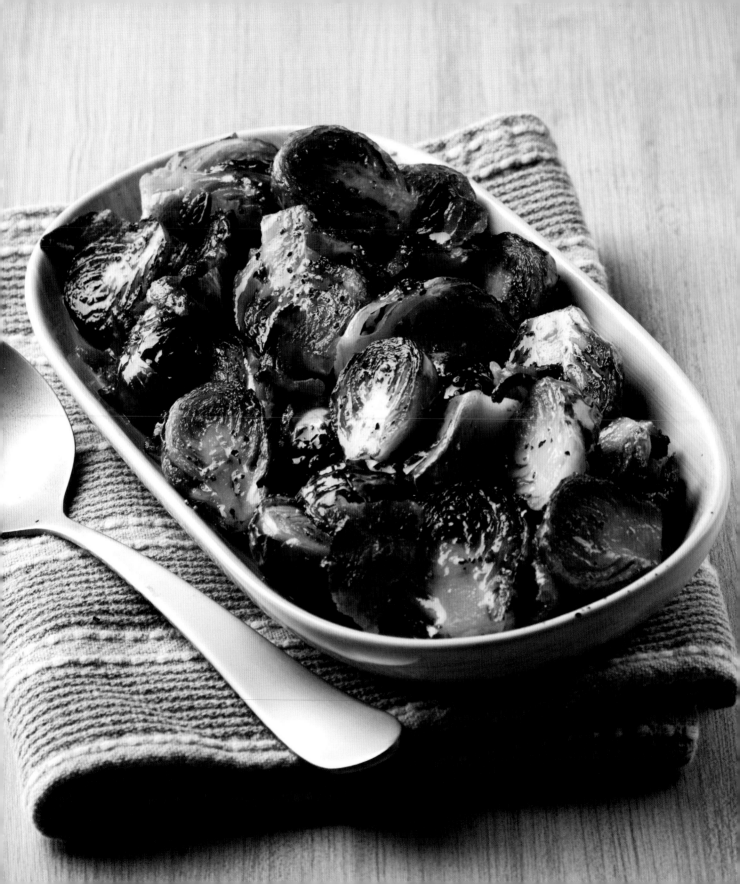

Vegetables and Sides

Brussels Sprouts with Bacon and Butter

MAKES 4 SERVINGS

1 Preheat oven to 375°F. Cook bacon in large cast iron skillet until almost crisp. Drain on paper towel-lined plate; set aside. Drain all but 1 tablespoon drippings.

2 Add brussels sprouts to skillet. Sprinkle with ¼ teaspoon salt and ¼ teaspoon pepper; toss to coat. Spread in skillet.

3 Roast 30 minutes or until brussels sprouts are browned and crispy, stirring every 10 minutes.

4 Add butter to skillet; stir until completely coated. Stir in bacon; season with additional salt and pepper.

6 slices thick-cut bacon, cut into ½-inch pieces

1½ pounds brussels sprouts (about 24 medium), halved

¼ teaspoon salt

¼ teaspoon black pepper

2 tablespoons butter, softened

Nutrients Per Serving (¼ of total recipe)

CALORIES 220 **TOTAL FAT** 15g **CARBS** 15g **NET CARBS** 8g
DIETARY FIBER 7g **PROTEIN** 10g

Zoodles in Tomato Sauce

MAKES 8 SERVINGS

3 teaspoons olive oil, divided

2 cloves garlic

1 tablespoon tomato paste

1 can (28 ounces) whole tomatoes, undrained

1 teaspoon dried oregano

½ teaspoon salt

2 large zucchini (about 16 ounces each), ends trimmed, cut into 3-inch pieces

¼ cup shredded Parmesan cheese

1 Heat 2 teaspoons oil in medium saucepan over medium heat. Add garlic; cook 1 minute or until fragrant but not browned. Stir in tomato paste; cook 30 seconds, stirring constantly. Add tomatoes with juice, oregano and salt; break up tomatoes with wooden spoon. Bring to a simmer. Reduce heat; cook 30 minutes or until thickened.

2 Meanwhile, spiral zucchini with fine spiral blade. Heat remaining 1 teaspoon oil in large skillet over medium-high heat. Add zucchini; cook 4 to 5 minutes or until tender, stirring frequently. Transfer to serving plates; top with tomato sauce and cheese.

Note: If you don't have a spiralizer, cut the zucchini into ribbons with a mandoline or sharp knife. Or buy 2 pounds of prepared zucchini noodles.

Nutrients Per Serving (⅛ of total recipe)

CALORIES 70   **TOTAL FAT** 3g   **CARBS** 8g   **NET CARBS** 5g
DIETARY FIBER 3g   **PROTEIN** 4g

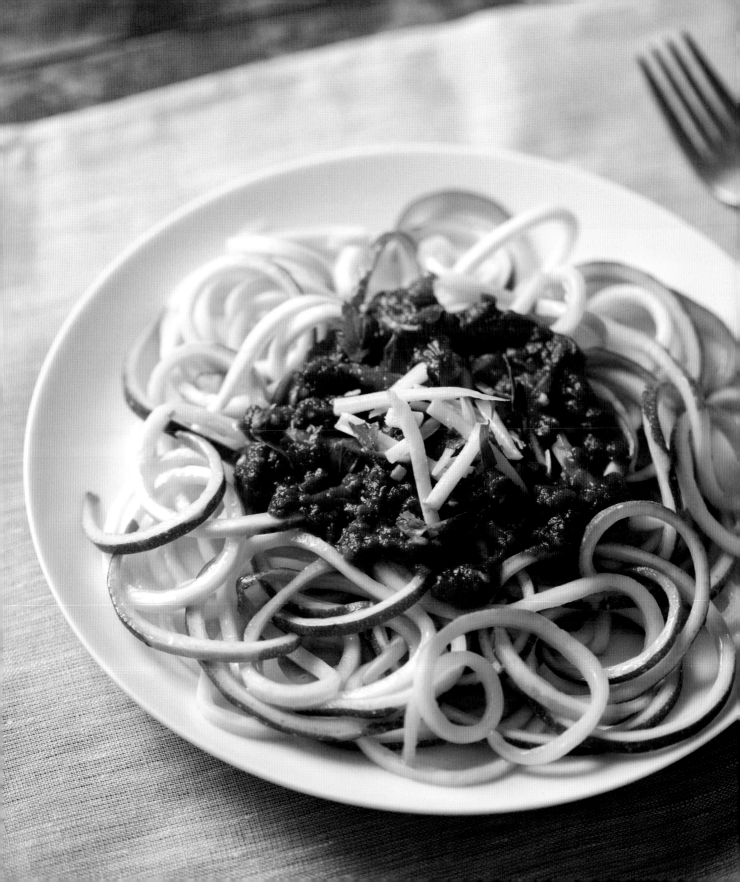

2 heads cauliflower (to equal 8 cups florets)

Salt

1 tablespoon butter or as needed

1 tablespoon half-and-half or whipping cream

Mashed Cauliflower

MAKES 6 SERVINGS

1 Break cauliflower into equal-size florets. Place in large saucepan; add about 2 inches of water and 1 teaspoon salt. Simmer over medium heat 20 to 25 minutes or until cauliflower is very tender and falling apart. (Check occasionally to make sure there is enough water to prevent burning; add water if necessary.) Drain well.

2 Place cauliflower in food processor or blender. Process until almost smooth. Add butter. Process until smooth, adding half-and-half as needed to reach desired consistency. Season with salt to taste.

Nutrients Per Serving (½ **cup**)

CALORIES 54   **TOTAL FAT** 2g   **CARBS** 7g   **NET CARBS** 4g
DIETARY FIBER 3g   **PROTEIN** 3g

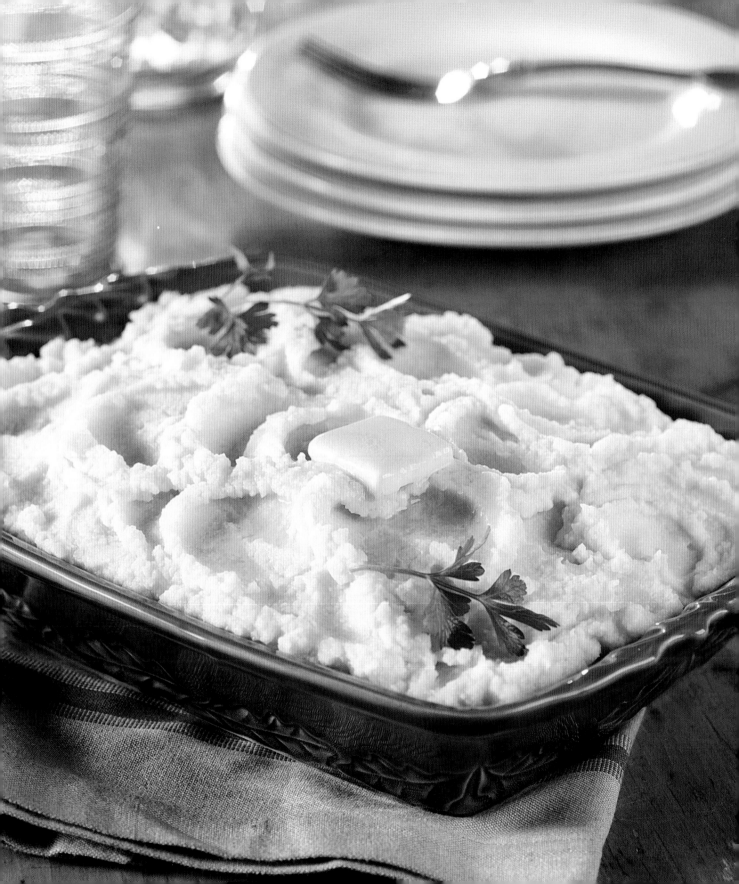

Red Cabbage with Bacon and Mushrooms

MAKES 6 SERVINGS

5 slices thick-cut bacon, chopped (about 8 ounces)

1 onion, chopped

1 package (8 ounces) cremini mushrooms, chopped (½-inch pieces)

¾ teaspoon dried thyme

½ medium red cabbage, cut into wedges, cored and then cut crosswise into ¼-inch slices (about 7 cups)

¾ teaspoon salt

¼ teaspoon black pepper

⅔ cup chicken broth

3 tablespoons cider vinegar

¼ cup chopped walnuts, toasted*

3 tablespoons chopped fresh parsley

*To toast walnuts, cook in small skillet over medium heat 4 to 5 minutes or until lightly browned, stirring frequently.

1 Cook bacon in large saucepan or skillet over medium-high heat until crisp. Remove to paper towel-lined plate.

2 Add onion to saucepan; cook and stir 5 minutes or until softened. Add mushrooms and thyme; cook about 6 minutes or until mushrooms begin to brown, stirring occasionally. Add cabbage, ¾ teaspoon salt and ¼ teaspoon pepper; cook about 7 minutes or until cabbage has wilted.

3 Stir in broth, vinegar and half of bacon; bring to a boil. Reduce heat to low; cook, uncovered, 15 to 20 minutes or until cabbage is tender.

4 Stir in walnuts and parsley; season with additional salt and pepper if necessary. Sprinkle with remaining bacon.

Nutrients Per Serving (⅙ of total recipe)

CALORIES 240 **TOTAL FAT** 14g **CARBS** 12g **NET CARBS** 9g **DIETARY FIBER** 3g **PROTEIN** 20g

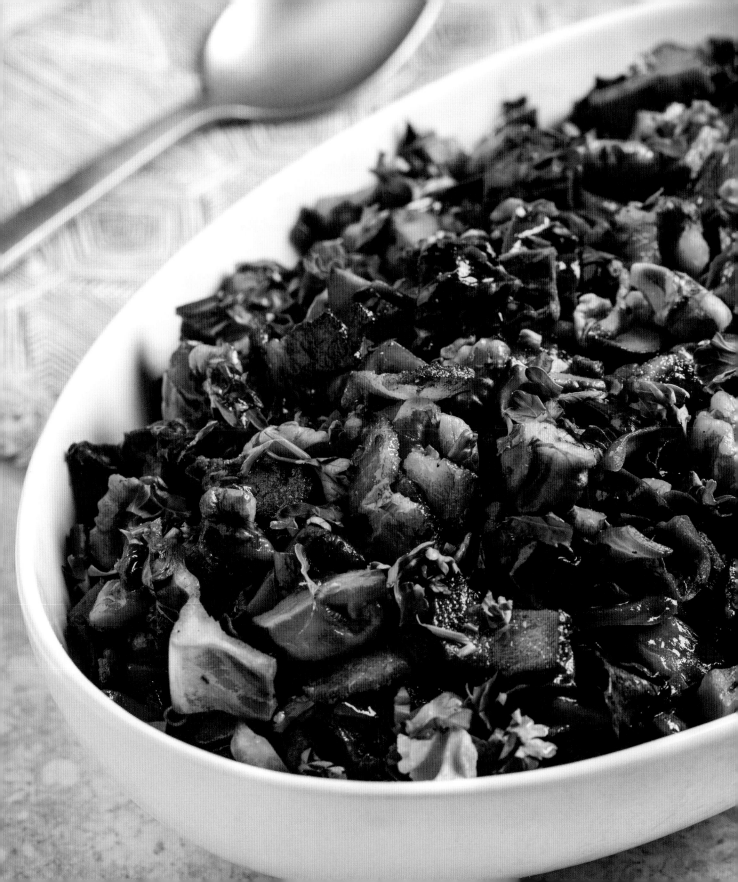

1 head cauliflower

1 tablespoon olive oil

3 tablespoons grated Parmesan cheese

2 tablespoons almond flour

½ teaspoon salt

½ teaspoon chopped fresh parsley

¼ teaspoon ground black pepper

Roasted Cauliflower

MAKES 4 SERVINGS

1 Preheat oven to 375°F. Spray large rimmed baking sheet with nonstick cooking spray.

2 Cut cauliflower into florets. Place in large bowl. Drizzle with oil. Sprinkle cheese, almond flour, salt, parsley and pepper over cauliflower; toss to coat. Spread cauliflower mixture on prepared baking sheet.

3 Bake 20 to 25 minutes or until cauliflower is browned and tender, stirring occasionally.

Nutrients Per Serving (¼ of total recipe)

CALORIES 110   **TOTAL FAT** 7g   **CARBS** 8g   **NET CARBS** 5g
DIETARY FIBER 3g   **PROTEIN** 6g

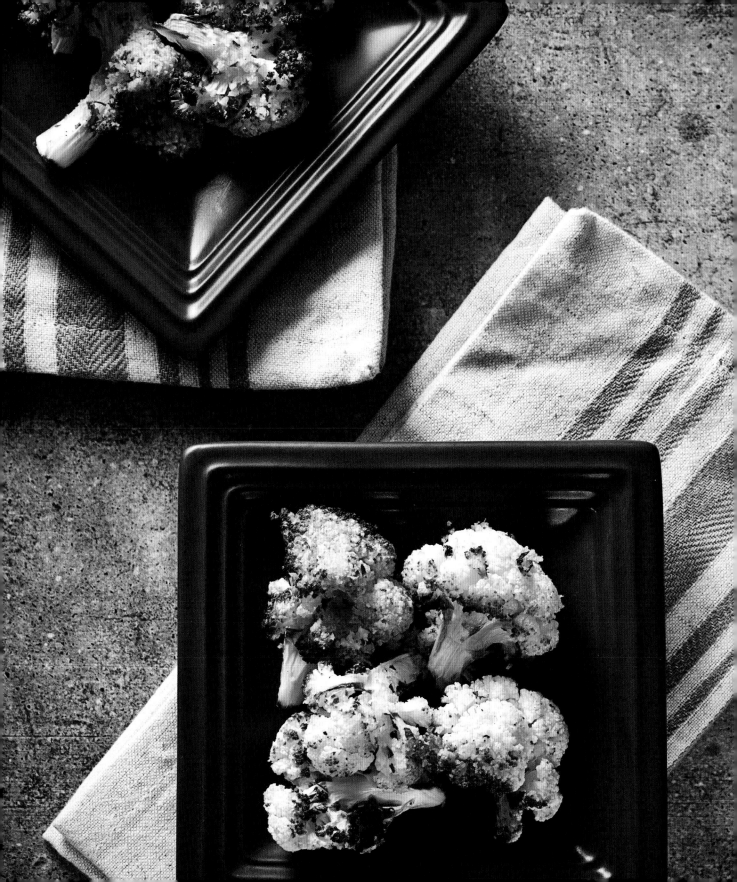

1 slice bacon, chopped

½ cup sliced shallots

1 package (4 ounces) sliced mixed exotic mushrooms *or* 2 cups sliced button mushrooms

10 cups (8 ounces) loosely packed torn fresh kale leaves (remove tough stems)*

2 tablespoons water

½ teaspoon black pepper

Look for 16-ounce bags of ready-to-cook fresh kale leaves in the produce section of the supermarket.

Sautéed Kale with Mushrooms and Bacon

MAKES 4 SERVINGS

1 Cook bacon in large skillet over medium heat 5 minutes. Add shallots; cook and stir 3 minutes. Add mushrooms; cook 8 minutes, stirring occasionally.

2 Add kale and water; cover and cook 5 minutes. Uncover; cook and stir 5 minutes or until kale is crisp-tender, stirring occasionally. Season with pepper.

Nutrients Per Serving (¼ of total recipe)

CALORIES 90 **TOTAL FAT** 4g **CARBS** 11g **NET CARBS** 8g
DIETARY FIBER 3g **PROTEIN** 4g

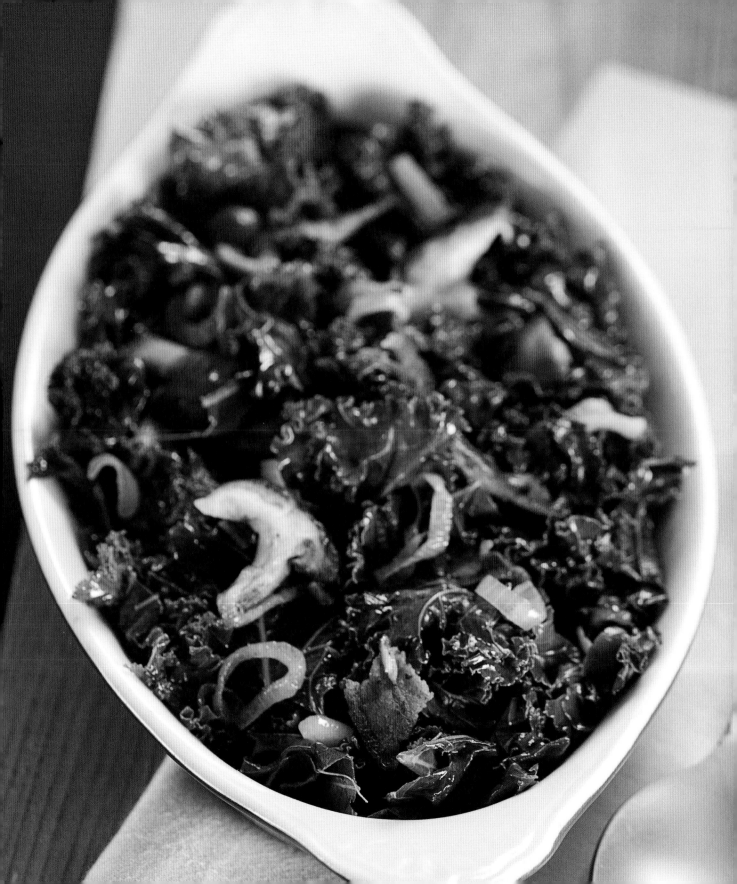

¼ cup thinly sliced sweet onion

1 block (8 ounces) feta cheese, thickly sliced crosswise

¼ cup thinly sliced green bell pepper

¼ cup thinly sliced red bell pepper

½ teaspoon dried oregano

¼ teaspoon garlic pepper or black pepper

Grilled Feta with Peppers
MAKES 8 SERVINGS

1 Spray 14-inch-long sheet of foil with nonstick cooking spray. Place onion in center of foil and top with cheese and bell peppers. Sprinkle with oregano and garlic pepper.

2 Bring two long sides of foil together above the food; fold down in a series of locked folds, allowing for heat circulation and expansion. Fold short ends up and over again. Press folds firmly to seal the foil packet. Place foil packet upside down on grid. Grill, covered, over high heat 15 minutes. Turn packet over; grill, covered, 15 minutes.

3 Open packet carefully and serve immediately.

Nutrients Per Serving (¼ of total recipe)
CALORIES 70 **TOTAL FAT** 5g **CARBS** 2g **NET CARBS** 2g
DIETARY FIBER 0g **PROTEIN** 5g

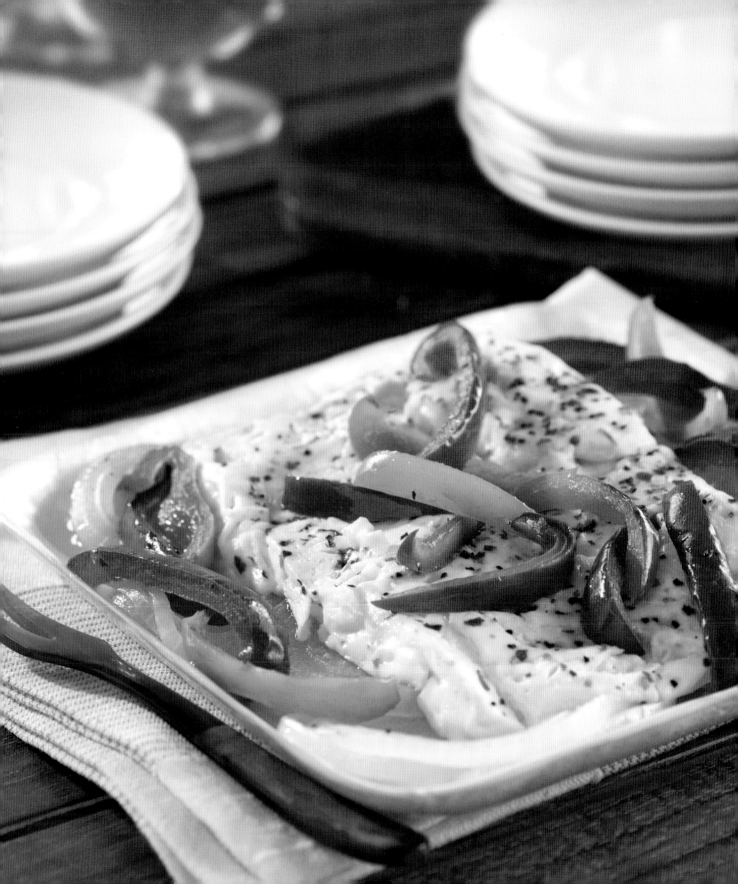

Kale with Caramelized Garlic
MAKES 6 SERVINGS

1½ pounds fresh kale, tough stems removed and discarded, leaves thinly sliced (16 cups)

2 cups water

1 tablespoon olive oil

8 cloves garlic, thinly sliced

1 teaspoon red wine vinegar

¼ teaspoon salt

⅛ to ¼ teaspoon red pepper flakes

1 Place kale and water in large saucepan; bring to a boil over medium-high heat. Cook, covered, about 6 to 8 minutes or until kale is tender but still bright green. Drain in colander.

2 Meanwhile, heat oil in large nonstick skillet over medium heat. Add garlic; cook and stir 2 to 4 minutes or until garlic is golden brown, being careful not to allow garlic to burn. Add kale, vinegar, salt and red pepper flakes; cook and stir until heated through.

Nutrients Per Serving (about 1 cup)

CALORIES 80 **TOTAL FAT** 4g **CARBS** 11g **NET CARBS** 7g
DIETARY FIBER 4g **PROTEIN** 5g

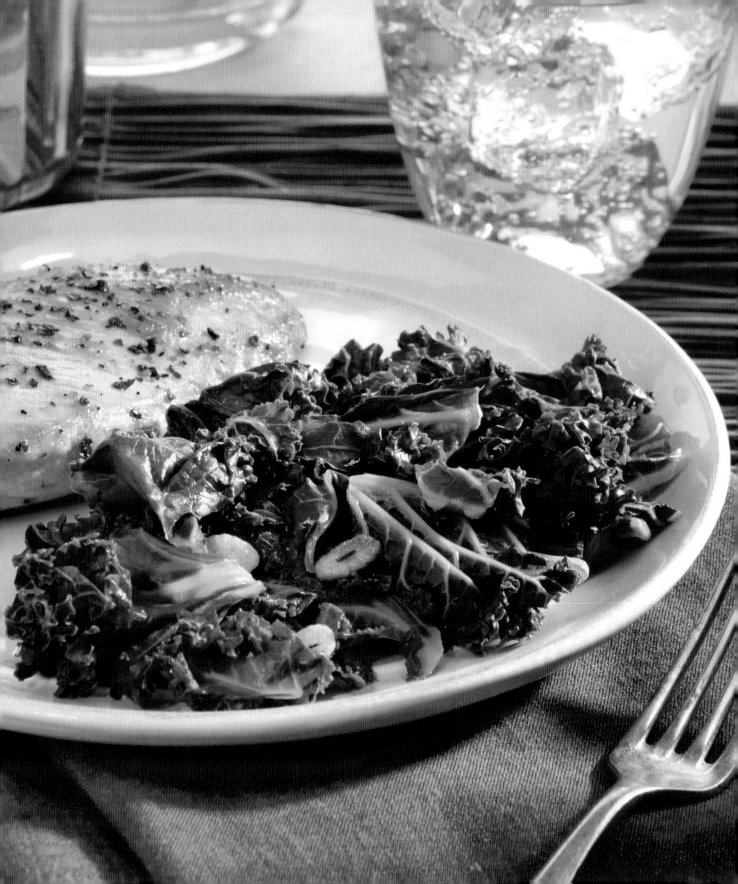

½ cup (1 stick) butter, divided

1 cup diced onion

1 large head cauliflower, broken into florets

½ cup water

Cauliflower with Onion Butter

MAKES 8 TO 10 SERVINGS

1 Melt ¼ cup butter in medium skillet over medium heat. Add onion; cook about 20 minutes or until onion is deep golden brown, stirring occasionally.

2 Meanwhile, place cauliflower and water in microwavable bowl. Microwave on HIGH 8 minutes or until crisp-tender; drain, if necessary.

3 Add remaining ¼ cup butter to skillet with onion; cook and stir until butter is melted. Pour over cauliflower; serve immediately.

Nutrients Per Serving (½ cup)

CALORIES 108   **TOTAL FAT** 11g   **CARBS** 2g   **NET CARBS** 1g
DIETARY FIBER 1g   **PROTEIN** 1g

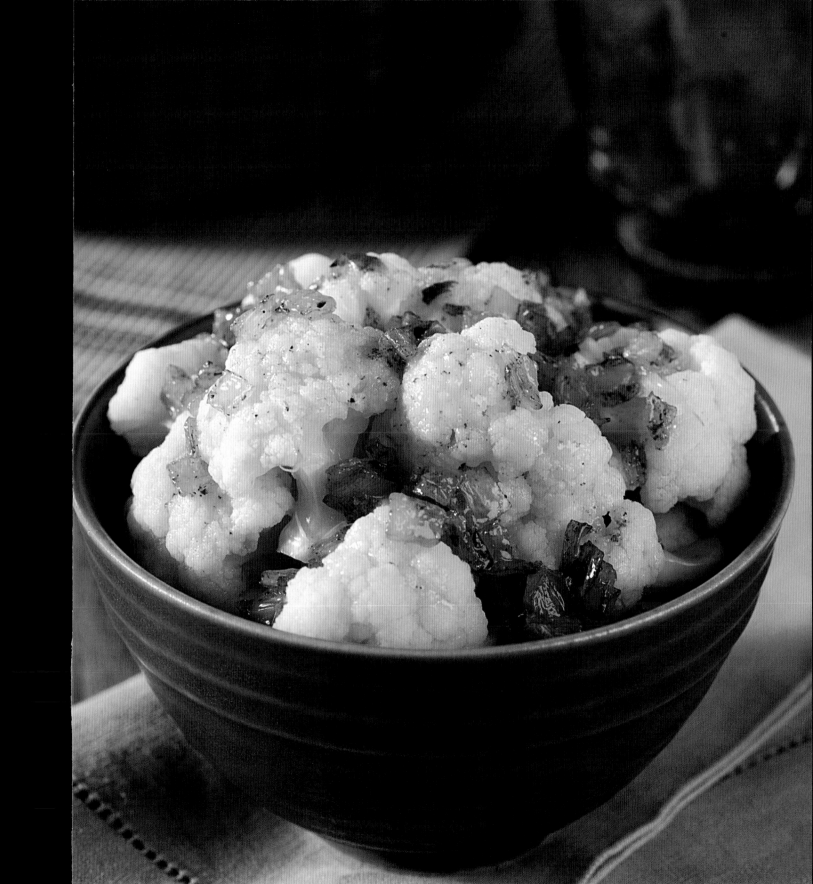

2 teaspoons olive oil

2 large zucchini or yellow squash, cut into ¼-inch slices (4 cups)

2 cloves garlic, minced

¼ teaspoon salt

¼ teaspoon black pepper

¼ cup thinly sliced basil

2 tablespoons grated Parmesan cheese

Quick Zucchini Parmesan

MAKES 4 SERVINGS

1 Heat oil in large nonstick skillet over medium heat. Add zucchini; cook and stir 2 minutes.

2 Add garlic, salt and pepper; cook 4 to 5 minutes or just until zucchini is tender. Top with basil and cheese.

Nutrients Per Serving (¾ cup)

CALORIES 50   **TOTAL FAT** 3g   **CARBS** 4g   **NET CARBS** 3g
DIETARY FIBER 1g   **PROTEIN** 2g

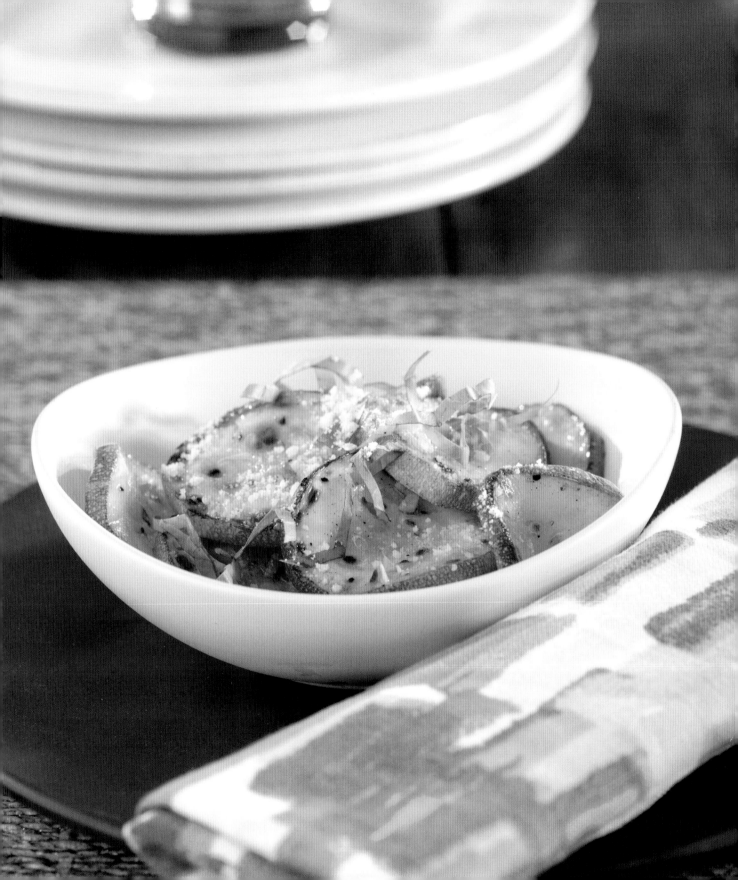

Cauliflower Tabbouleh

MAKES 6 SERVINGS

2 heads cauliflower
(12 ounces each),
cut into florets

3 tablespoons olive oil,
divided

1 teaspoon curry
powder

1 small bunch fresh
Italian parsley

1 medium onion, finely
chopped (¾ cup)

½ seedless cucumber,
chopped (1½ cups)

1 cup chopped ripe
tomato *or* 1 can
(about 14 ounces)
diced tomatoes,
well drained

⅓ cup fresh lemon juice

½ teaspoon salt

½ teaspoon black
pepper

1 Place cauliflower in food processor or blender; pulse 1 minute or until chopped into uniform granules.

2 Heat 1 tablespoon oil in large nonstick skillet over medium-high heat. Add curry powder; cook until sizzling. Add cauliflower; stir-fry about 10 minutes or until cooked through. Remove from heat and cool.

3 Meanwhile, rinse parsley, trim and discard large stems. Place parsley sprigs in food processor; pulse 10 to 20 seconds to chop.

4 Combine cauliflower mixture, parsley, onion, cucumber and tomato in large bowl. Whisk remaining 2 tablespoons oil, lemon juice, salt and pepper in small bowl. Pour over cauliflower mixture; toss well. Serve at room temperature or chilled.

Nutrients Per Serving (1 cup)

CALORIES 114   **TOTAL FAT** 7g   **CARBS** 12g   **NET CARBS** 8g
DIETARY FIBER 4g   **PROTEIN** 3g

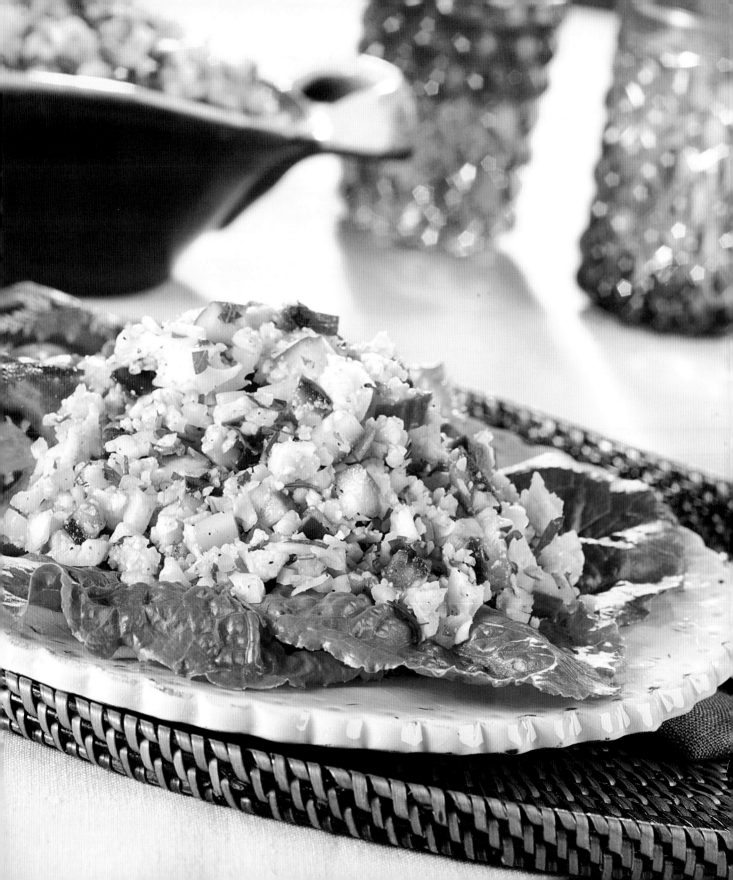

3 packages (10 ounces each) frozen chopped spinach

1 tablespoon canola oil

1 onion, chopped

1 clove garlic, minced

2 Anaheim chiles, toasted, peeled and minced

3 fresh tomatillos, toasted,* husks removed and chopped

6 tablespoons sour cream (optional)

To toast fresh tomatillos, preheat heavy frying pan over medium heat. Leaving papery husks on, toast tomatillos, turning often, about 10 minutes or until husks are brown and interior flesh is soft. Remove from heat. When cool enough to handle, remove and discard husks.

Mexican-Style Spinach
MAKES 6 SERVINGS

Slow Cooker Directions

1 Place frozen spinach in slow cooker.

2 Heat oil in large skillet over medium heat. Add onion and garlic; cook and stir about 5 minutes or until onion is softened. Add chiles and tomatillos; cook and stir 2 minutes. Transfer mixture to slow cooker. Cover; cook on LOW 4 to 6 hours. Stir before serving. Top with dollops of sour cream, if desired.

Substitution: Two pounds of fresh spinach (about 5 quarts) or other greens such as bagged baby spinach or mixed wild greens can be substituted for the frozen spinach. If using fresh bundled spinach, be sure to trim the stems and thoroughly wash the leaves in several changes of water to remove any sand before chopping.

Nutrients Per Serving (1 cup spinach)
CALORIES 73　**TOTAL FAT** 3g　**CARBS** 10g　**NET CARBS** 5g
DIETARY FIBER 5g　**PROTEIN** 5g

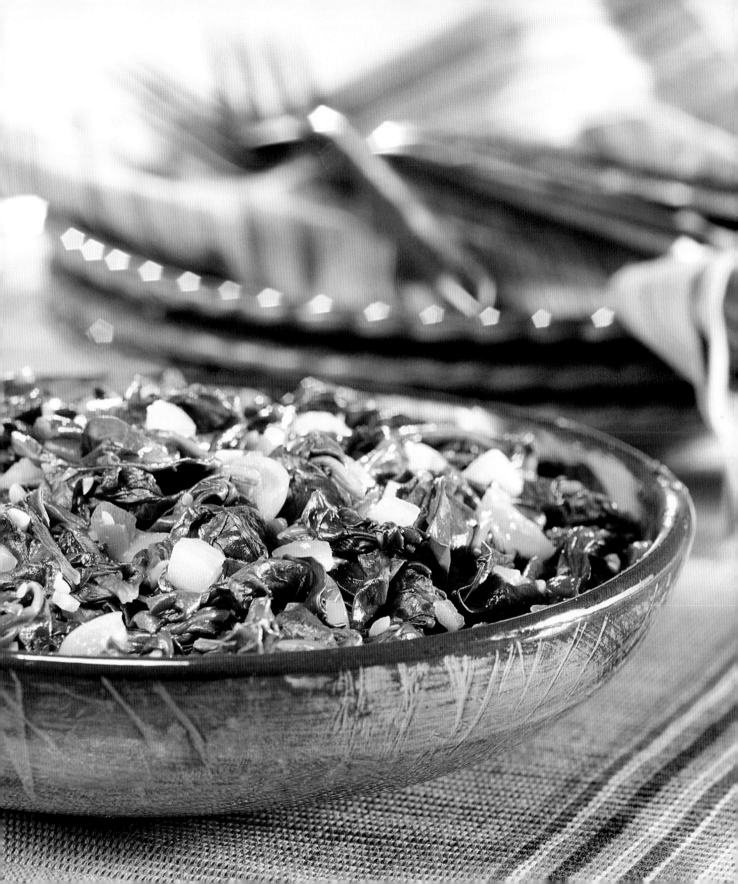

1 cup water

1 pound asparagus, trimmed

1 package (3½ ounces) goat cheese

¾ cup chicken broth

¼ cup dry white wine

2 cloves garlic, minced

2 tablespoons chopped fresh chives

Asparagus with Goat Cheese Sauce
MAKES 4 SERVINGS

1 Bring water to a boil in large skillet. Add asparagus; cover and steam 3 to 5 minutes or until crisp-tender. Transfer to serving plate.

2 Meanwhile for sauce, mash cheese in medium nonstick skillet; stir in broth, wine and garlic. Simmer over medium heat 8 to 10 minutes or until desired thickness, stirring frequently. Fold in chives; serve immediately over asparagus.

Nutrients Per Serving
(¼ **pound asparagus and** ¼ **cup sauce)**

CALORIES 135   **TOTAL FAT** 8g   **CARBS** 7g   **NET CARBS** 5g

DIETARY FIBER 2g   **PROTEIN** 8g

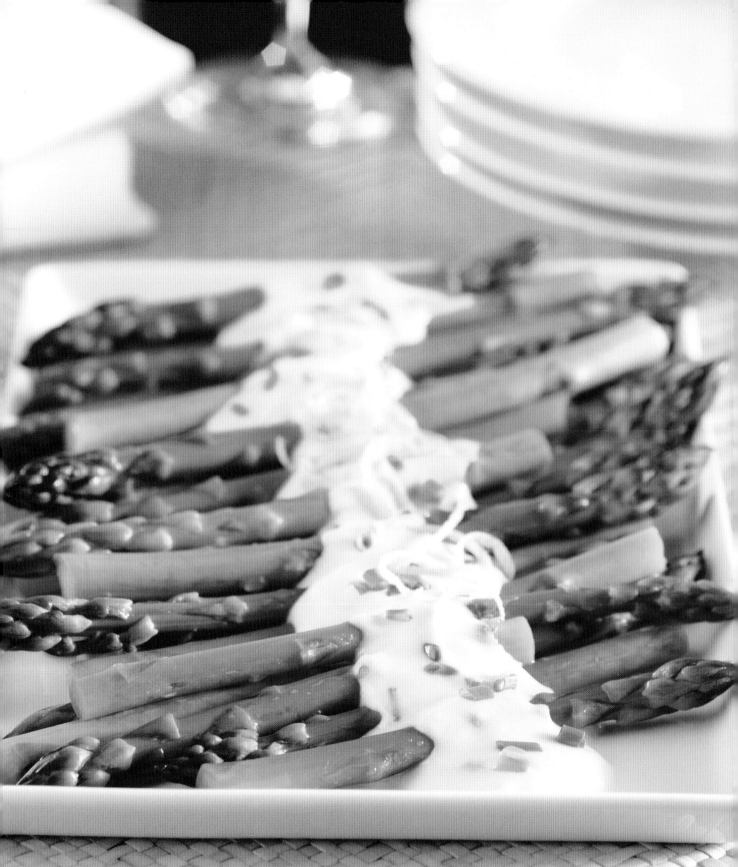

Creamy Parmesan Spinach

MAKES 6 SERVINGS

2 tablespoons butter, divided

1 cup finely chopped yellow onion

2 packages (9 ounces each) fresh spinach, divided

3 ounces cream cheese, cut into pieces

½ teaspoon garlic powder

¼ teaspoon ground nutmeg

¼ teaspoon black pepper

⅛ teaspoon salt

2 tablespoons grated Parmesan, pecorino or Monterey Jack cheese

1 Melt 1 tablespoon butter in large skillet over medium-high heat. Add onion; cook and stir 4 minutes or until translucent.

2 Add 1 package of spinach; cook and stir 2 minutes or just until wilted. Transfer spinach mixture to medium bowl. Repeat with remaining 1 tablespoon butter and spinach.

3 Return reserved spinach to skillet. Add cream cheese, garlic powder, nutmeg, pepper and salt; cook and stir until cream cheese has completely melted.

4 Sprinkle with Parmesan cheese just before serving.

Variation: For a thinner consistency, add 2 to 3 tablespoons milk before adding the Parmesan cheese.

Nutrients Per Serving (½ cup)

CALORIES 130   **TOTAL FAT** 10g   **CARBS** 7g   **NET CARBS** 5g
DIETARY FIBER 2g   **PROTEIN** 5g

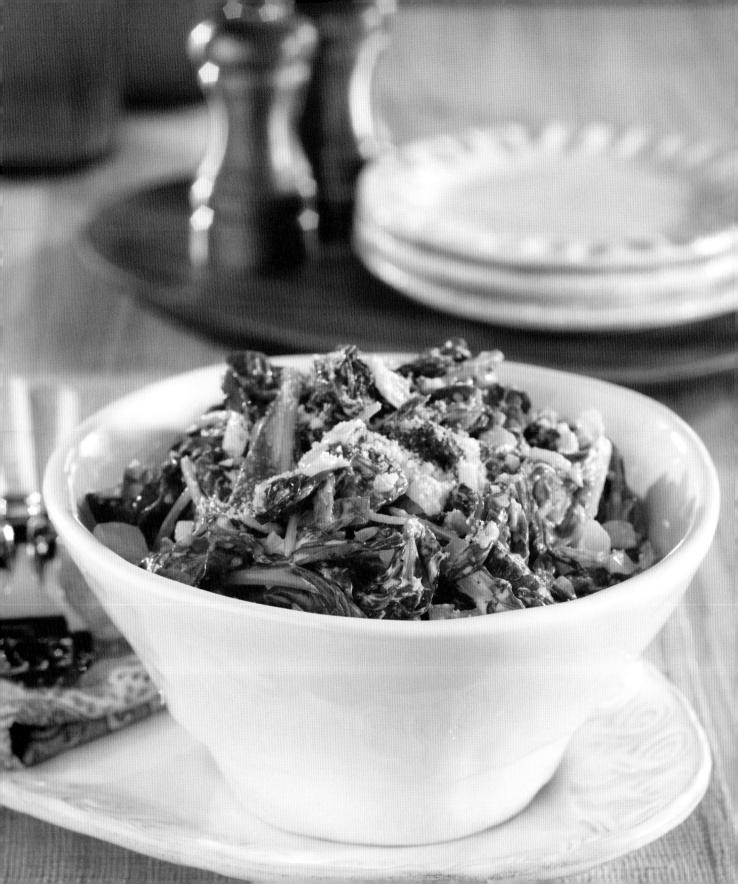

¼ cup (½ stick) butter

¼ cup almond flour

1½ cups milk, warmed to room temperature

¼ teaspoon salt

¼ teaspoon ground red pepper

⅛ teaspoon black pepper

6 eggs, separated

1 cup (4 ounces) shredded Cheddar cheese

Pinch cream of tartar (optional)

Cheese Soufflé

MAKES 4 SERVINGS

1 Preheat oven to 375°F. Grease four 2-cup soufflé dishes or one 2-quart soufflé dish.

2 Melt butter in large saucepan over medium-low heat. Add almond flour; whisk 2 minutes or until mixture just begins to color. Gradually whisk in milk. Add salt, red pepper and black pepper; whisk until mixture comes to a boil and thickens. Remove from heat. Stir in egg yolks, one at a time, and cheese.

3 Beat egg whites and cream of tartar in large bowl with electric mixer at high speed until stiff peaks form.

4 Gently fold egg whites into cheese mixture until almost combined. (Some streaks of white should remain.) Transfer mixture to prepared dishes.

5 Bake small soufflés about 20 minutes (30 to 40 minutes for large soufflé) or until puffed and browned and tester inserted into center comes out moist but clean. Serve immediately.

Nutrients Per Serving (¼ of total recipe)

CALORIES 380 **TOTAL FAT** 30g **CARBS** 7g **NET CARBS** 6g
DIETARY FIBER 1g **PROTEIN** 21g

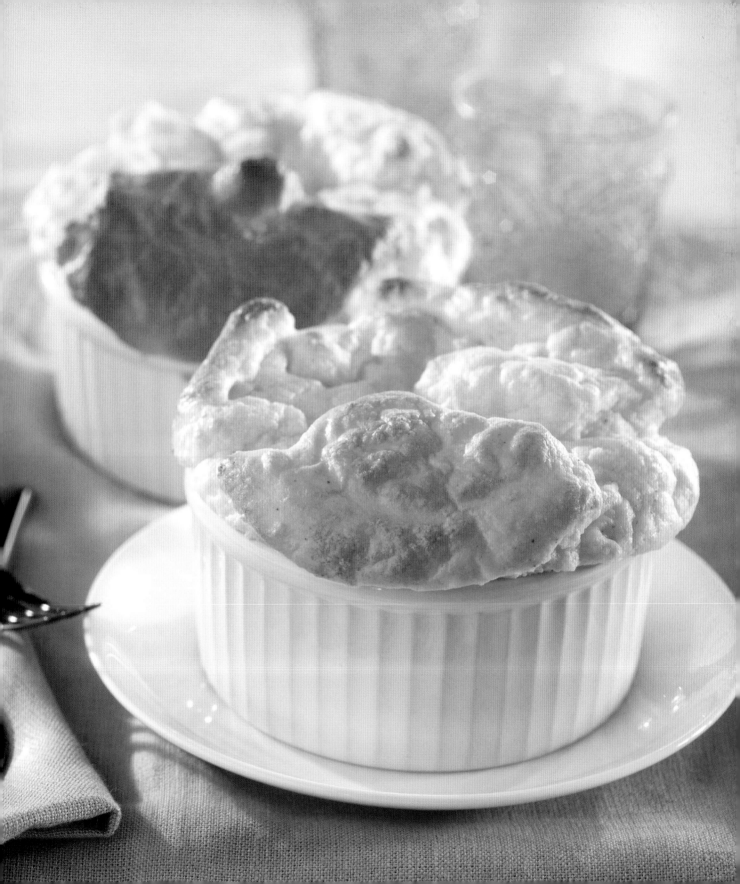

2 heads cauliflower, cut into florets (8 cups)

2 tablespoons olive oil

1 teaspoon salt

¼ cup (½ stick) butter, cut into small pieces

¼ cup milk

½ cup chopped green onions, divided

1 cup (4 ounces) shredded Cheddar cheese, divided

4 ounces bacon, crisp cooked and crumbled

½ cup chopped tomatoes

Sour cream

Twice Baked Loaded Cauliflower

MAKES 8 SERVINGS (4 CUPS MASHED CAULIFLOWER)

1 Preheat oven to 425°F. Divide cauliflower between two 13×9-inch baking pans. Drizzle each with 1 tablespoon oil and sprinkle each with ½ teaspoon salt. Roast 40 minutes, stirring cauliflower and rotating pans once. *Reduce oven temperature to 375°F.*

2 Transfer cauliflower to food processor; add butter and milk. Process 1 to 2 minutes or until very smooth and fluffy. Stir in half of green onions and ½ cup cheese. Divide mixture among eight ramekins. Sprinkle with remaining cheese and bacon.

3 Bake 10 to 15 minutes or until cheese is melted and browned around edge and cauliflower is heated through. Top with remaining green onions, tomatoes and sour cream.

Nutrients Per Serving
(½ cup cauliflower with ¼ of toppings)

CALORIES 250 **TOTAL FAT** 18g **CARBS** 12g **NET CARBS** 7g
DIETARY FIBER 5g **PROTEIN** 13g

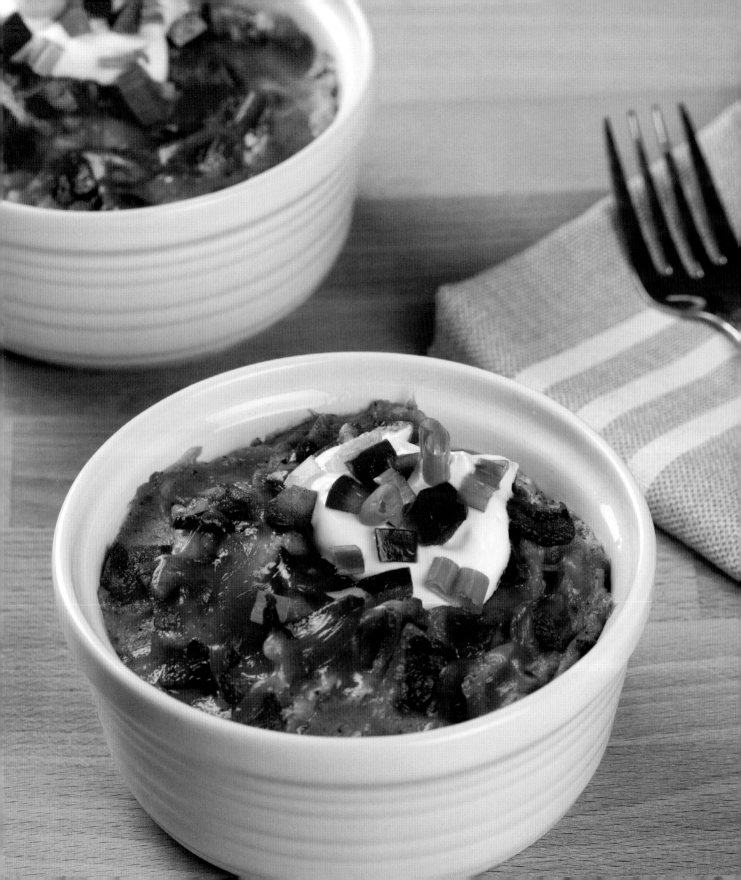

Spinach Artichoke Gratin

MAKES 6 SERVINGS

2 cups (16 ounces) cottage cheese

2 eggs

4½ tablespoons grated Parmesan cheese, divided

1 tablespoon lemon juice

⅛ teaspoon black pepper

⅛ teaspoon ground nutmeg

2 packages (10 ounces each) frozen chopped spinach, thawed

⅓ cup thinly sliced green onions

1 package (10 ounces) frozen artichoke hearts, thawed and halved

1 Preheat oven to 375°F. Spray 1½-quart baking dish with nonstick cooking spray.

2 Combine cottage cheese, eggs, 3 tablespoons Parmesan cheese, lemon juice, pepper and nutmeg in food processor or blender; process until smooth.

3 Squeeze moisture from spinach. Combine spinach, cottage cheese mixture and green onions in large bowl; mix well. Spread half of mixture in prepared baking dish.

4 Pat artichokes dry with paper towels; place in single layer over spinach mixture. Sprinkle with remaining 1½ tablespoons Parmesan cheese. Cover with remaining spinach mixture.

5 Cover and bake 25 minutes.

Nutrients Per Serving (1 cup)

CALORIES 170   **TOTAL FAT** 7g   **CARBS** 12g   **NET CARBS** 5g
DIETARY FIBER 7g   **PROTEIN** 18g

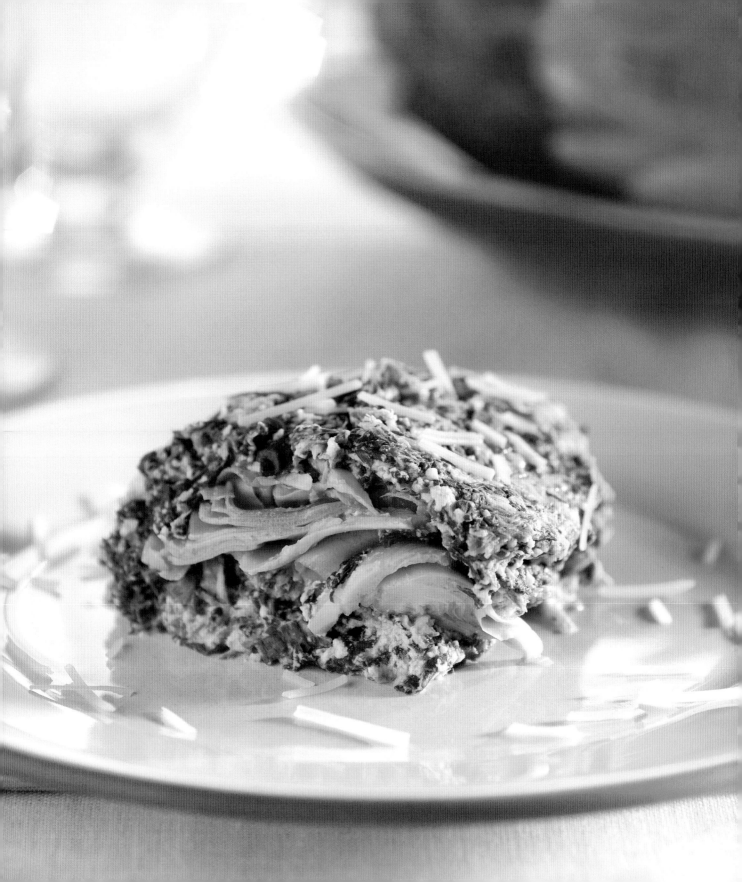

1 large bunch kale
(about 1 pound)

1 to 2 tablespoons
olive oil

1 teaspoon garlic salt
or other seasoned
salt

Kale Chips
MAKES 6 SERVINGS

1 Preheat oven to 350°F. Line baking sheets with
parchment paper.

2 Wash kale and pat dry with paper towels. Remove
center ribs and stems; discard. Cut leaves into 2- to
3-inch-wide pieces.

3 Combine leaves, oil and garlic salt in large bowl; toss
to coat. Spread onto prepared baking sheets.

4 Bake 10 to 15 minutes or until edges are lightly browned
and leaves are crisp.* Cool completely on baking sheets.
Store in airtight container.

*If the leaves are lightly browned but not crisp, turn oven off and
let chips stand in oven until crisp, about 10 minutes. Do not keep
the oven on as the chips will burn easily.*

Nutrients Per Serving (⅙ of total recipe)
CALORIES 60 **TOTAL FAT** 3g **CARBS** 7g **NET CARBS** 4g
DIETARY FIBER 3g **PROTEIN** 3g

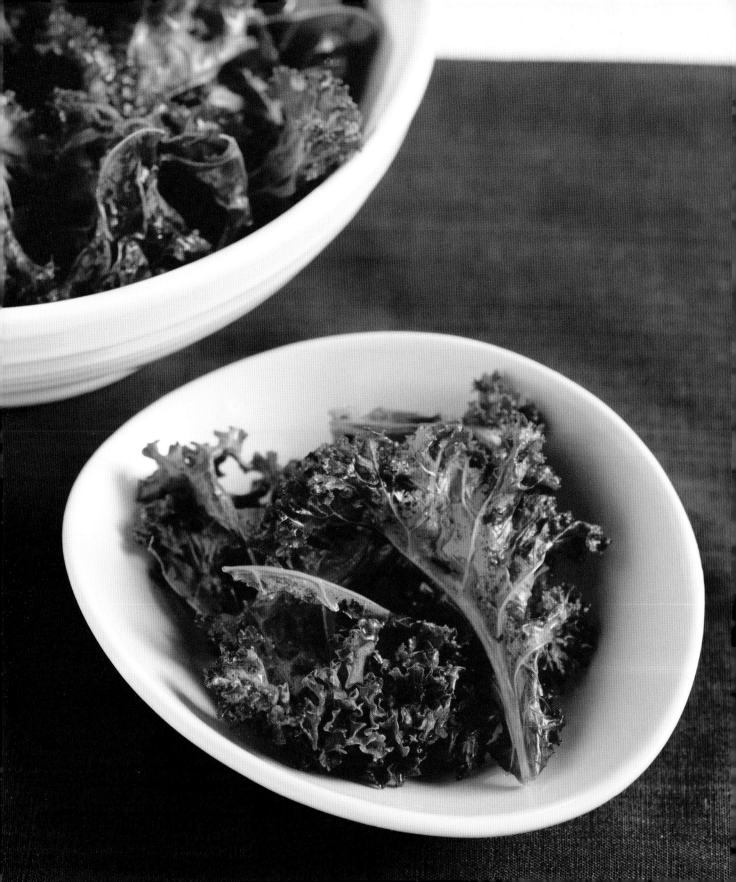

Index

Index

Metric Conversion Chart

VOLUME MEASUREMENTS (dry)

1/8 teaspoon = 0.5 mL
1/4 teaspoon = 1 mL
1/2 teaspoon = 2 mL
3/4 teaspoon = 4 mL
1 teaspoon = 5 mL
1 tablespoon = 15 mL
2 tablespoons = 30 mL
1/4 cup = 60 mL
1/3 cup = 75 mL
1/2 cup = 125 mL
2/3 cup = 150 mL
3/4 cup = 175 mL
1 cup = 250 mL
2 cups = 1 pint = 500 mL
3 cups = 750 mL
4 cups = 1 quart = 1 L

VOLUME MEASUREMENTS (fluid)

1 fluid ounce (2 tablespoons) = 30 mL
4 fluid ounces (1/2 cup) = 125 mL
8 fluid ounces (1 cup) = 250 mL
12 fluid ounces (1 1/2 cups) = 375 mL
16 fluid ounces (2 cups) = 500 mL

WEIGHTS (mass)

1/2 ounce = 15 g
1 ounce = 30 g
3 ounces = 90 g
4 ounces = 120 g
8 ounces = 225 g
10 ounces = 285 g
12 ounces = 360 g
16 ounces = 1 pound = 450 g

DIMENSIONS

1/16 inch = 2 mm
1/8 inch = 3 mm
1/4 inch = 6 mm
1/2 inch = 1.5 cm
3/4 inch = 2 cm
1 inch = 2.5 cm

OVEN TEMPERATURES

250°F = 120°C
275°F = 140°C
300°F = 150°C
325°F = 160°C
350°F = 180°C
375°F = 190°C
400°F = 200°C
425°F = 220°C
450°F = 230°C

BAKING PAN SIZES

Utensil	Size in Inches/Quarts	Metric Volume	Size in Centimeters
Baking or Cake Pan (square or rectangular)	8×8×2	2 L	20×20×5
	9×9×2	2.5 L	23×23×5
	12×8×2	3 L	30×20×5
	13×9×2	3.5 L	33×23×5
Loaf Pan	8×4×3	1.5 L	20×10×7
	9×5×3	2 L	23×13×7
Round Layer Cake Pan	8×1½	1.2 L	20×4
	9×1½	1.5 L	23×4
Pie Plate	8×1¼	750 mL	20×3
	9×1¼	1 L	23×3
Baking Dish or Casserole	1 quart	1 L	—
	1½ quart	1.5 L	—
	2 quart	2 L	—